Inside the Mayo Clinic

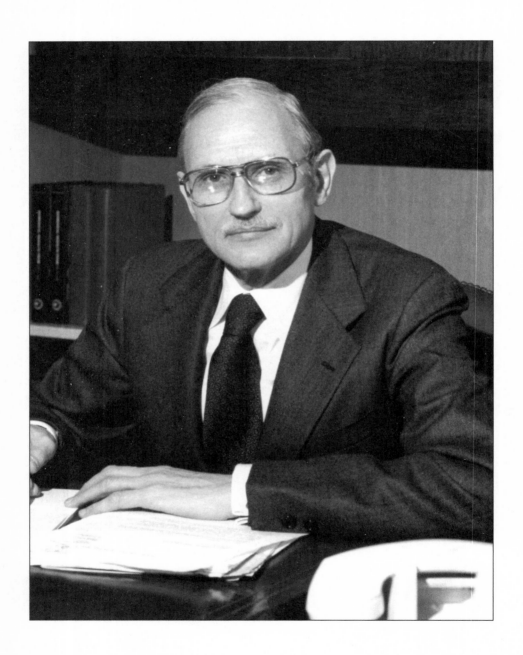

Inside the Mayo Clinic

a memoir

John T. Shepherd, M.D.

FOREWORD BY

WALTER F. MONDALE

AFTON HISTORICAL SOCIETY PRESS
AFTON, MINNESOTA

First edition

Editing by Michele Hodgson
Cover and book design by Mary Susan Oleson
Printed by Pettit Network, Inc., Afton, Minnesota

Library of Congress Cataloging-in-Publication Data
Shepherd, John T. (John Thompson), 1919-
Inside the Mayo clinic : a memoir / John T. Shepherd.—1st ed.
p. cm.
Includes index.
ISBN 1-890434-61-2
1. Mayo Clinic—History. 2. Shepherd, John T. (John Thompson), 1919-
I. Title.

RA982.R56 M48 2003
362.11'09776'155--dc22
2003017401

Printed in China

Afton Historical Society Press publishes exceptional books on regional subjects.

W. Duncan MacMillan
President

Patricia Condon Johnston
Publisher

Afton Historical Society Press
P.O. Box 100, Afton, MN 55001
(651) 436-8443 or (800) 436-8443

E-mail: aftonpress@aftonpress.com
www.aftonpress.com

Contents

Foreword

Before I became U.S. ambassador to Japan in 1993, I was a member of the Mayo Clinic and Foundation's board of trustees for four years. Upon my return to Minnesota in 1997, I rejoined the board, serving another four years. During both stints I gained not only an intimate knowledge of the history of the Mayo Clinic—whose roots in Rochester, Minnesota, reach back to the Civil War and frontier surgeon William Worrall Mayo—but also an appreciation of its pioneering approach to group medical practice. That approach emphasizes research and education as equal parts of its mission to provide the best possible care to patients. That approach also ensures that Mayo physicians won't personally profit from caring for the sick. Decades ago, W. W. Mayo's sons, Dr. Charles H. Mayo and Dr. William J. Mayo, put their colleagues on salary, a policy that continues to this day. Mayo doctors also receive no bonuses, have no profit-sharing privileges, and have no tenure. There's no reward for seeing more patients in less time. In this age of HMOs the Mayo method of practicing medicine is, to my mind, an ideal model to follow in reforming our country's troubled health care system. Indeed, I believe that the Mayo medical system is the best in the world.

One of the great players in the remarkable history of the Mayo Clinic is Dr. John Shepherd, who for fifty years has worked within Mayo's ideal model of research, education, and medical practice as a scientist, teacher, and administrator. He is an old friend with whom I have worked over the years. *Inside the Mayo Clinic* describes his personal recollections of half a century of change and growth and contribution at the world's best-known medical practice. John's career at the clinic began in 1953, when he left his native Ireland to come to Mayo on sabbatical from Queen's University of Belfast. He returned permanently to Rochester in 1957 to join Mayo's staff as a medical scientist in the physiology department, which he chaired for eight years.

As a researcher, John conducted studies on the human cardiovascular system. In the process he trained forty research fellows, who today occupy positions of responsibility and prominence in clinics, hospitals, and medical schools throughout the world. He also became the clinic's first director for research in 1969, not to mention president of the American Heart Association, a member of a U.S. medical delegation to the Soviet Union, and a research fraud investigator for the National Institutes of Health. As a member of NASA's Life Sciences Advisory Board, he had a front-row seat at mission control as America sent its first astronauts into space.

As an educator, John became Mayo's director for education in 1977 and as such contributed to the creation of the Mayo Medical School. As the fledgling school's second dean, he successfully pushed to make it a separate degree-granting institution from the University of Minnesota.

John also contributed significantly to Mayo's medical practice, not only through his hands-on research but also as an administrator serving the clinic's board of governors, board of trustees, and board of development. As a Mayo governor, he and his colleagues laid the groundwork for the Mayo Clinics of Jacksonville, Florida, and Scottsdale, Arizona. As a Mayo trustee, he helped guide the clinic's continuing mission, working side by side with the likes of future Supreme Court Justice Warren Burger and former president Lyndon Johnson. As chair of the board of development, John helped raise funds through such major benefactors as Barbara Woodward Lips (her bequest of $127.9 million is the largest gift to an academic medical center in American history) and Leslie and Susan Gonda, whose namesake facility, the Gonda Building, is the largest construction project to date at the Rochester clinic. Such funds have led to astonishing growth in research, educational, and medical facilities at Jacksonville and Phoenix as well.

John retired from the Mayo Clinic in 1990, but even at the age of eighty-four continues his involvement in research as chair of the Mayo Committee on the Application of Gene Therapy, applying his knowledge, perspective, and experience to the challenges of genetic research and treatments. Throughout his distinguished career he has received a long list of awards and honors, the latest bestowed in June 2003 when he became an honorary fellow of the Royal College of Physicians of Ireland.

John is one of Minnesota's most respected citizens, and he and his wife, Marion, with whom I've also worked on various nonprofit activities, particularly during her time as director of the Minneapolis Foundation, are one of Minnesota's truly remarkable couples.

Inside the Mayo Clinic recollects John Shepherd's career against the dynamic backdrop of the internationally renowned facility during its decades of greatest growth. It's a fascinating story of his experiences at a unique institution that is both a local legend and an international treasure.

Walter F. Mondale

Acknowledgments

Although I am the author of several medical texts, writing a memoir of my fifty years as a scientist, educator, and administrator at the Mayo Clinic has been a new and exciting adventure. For sharing that excitement, and for her careful and caring guidance in bringing this book to fruition, I am most grateful to Patricia Johnston, publisher of Afton Historical Society Press. For her hard work and enthusiasm as my editor, great appreciation goes as well to Michele Hodgson.

Each and every member of my family and my wife's family championed my efforts on this project. I owe heartfelt thanks to my children, Dr. Gillian Shepherd and Dr. Roger Shepherd, and to their spouses, Eduardo Mestre and Wendy Shepherd, for their love and encouragement. I am especially thankful as well to Nancy Etzwiler and to her husband, Dan O'Neill, who kindly introduced me to Patricia at Afton Press, and to my wife's three other children and their spouses: Drs. Lisa Etzwiler and Randall Clary; Diane Etzwiler and Robert Thallon; and David Etzwiler and Sarah Truesdell. My cousin, Eleanor Cameron, deserves my appreciation for verifying the Shepherd family history contained in my manuscript, and if he were alive, I would surely thank my brother Fred, whose gift to me of Helen Clapesattle's *The Doctors Mayo* back in 1946 first inspired me to pursue a future at the renowned clinic.

Two Mayo colleagues in particular, Dr. Joseph Kiely and Dr. Oliver Beahrs, offered kind and continuing support over the course of several years as I strived to capture the varied aspects of Mayo history. Friends and colleagues Colum and Una Gorman, Michael and Margaret O'Sullivan, and Daniel and Ruth Connally gave much encouragement as well. For her unflagging assistance to me as a Mayo emeritus staff member, I sincerely thank my secretary, Jacqueline Goetzman.

ACKNOWLEDGMENTS

For generously contributing the foreword that graces this memoir, I owe a particular debt of gratitude to former Mayo trustee, U.S. senator, vice president, and U.S. ambassador, the Honorable Walter F. Mondale.

For her patience and devotion during the time I was writing my reminiscences, I lovingly thank my wife, Marion Etzwiler Shepherd. Her advice and ideas helped immeasurably as I followed my dream of recording the events leading to my arrival at the Mayo Clinic, and the extraordinary personal and professional events that followed.

Many of the photos that appear in this book come from my personal files, but for the use of stock institutional photos, I would like to acknowledge the Mayo Clinic.

I am thankful, of course, for the opportunities and satisfaction the field of medicine has given me and my family. Yet my greatest measure of gratitude goes to the Mayo Clinic and Foundation, which has allowed me to contribute both to the practice and to my profession in ways I likely never could have someplace else. Although its primary site is located in a relatively small Minnesota community, Mayo is known the world over for its leadership in medicine, and I have been blessed to work beside many distinguished colleagues, fellows, and benefactors. It is my hope that, by reading my recollections of my half century at Mayo, new members of its staff will fully appreciate the uniqueness of this institution and endeavor to preserve the principles of William Worrall Mayo and his sons, Will and Charlie, that have guided and governed this remarkable clinic since its founding.

1

the road to Mayo

In the postwar summer of 1946, I was newly married and newly graduated from medical school, with intentions of becoming a physician like my uncle and brothers before me. That fall, I was set to begin my postgraduate training at Queen's University in Belfast, but for the moment I was happily vacationing with my bride and family in County Donegal off the northwest coast of my native Ireland. During that idyllic August, I read The Doctors Mayo, *a gift from my brother Fred. Written by Helen Clapesattle, the book told of the unlikely birth of a renowned medical institution, whose legacy of caring for patients began in an obscure town in southeastern Minnesota during the Civil War with frontier surgeon William Worrall Mayo. The impact that his intriguing story, and that of his famous sons, had on me was nothing less than life-changing. By the time I finished the book, I knew that I must someday see this unique place for myself.*

My fascination with Mayo was renewed when, in 1953, I had the chance to spend a sabbatical year in Rochester, Minnesota, researching heart disease in the clinic's physiology department. And though I turned down Mayo when it first called in 1955 to offer me a staff position, I accepted its second invitation one year later. Like hundreds of thousands of Irish immigrants in centuries past, I set sail for America with dreams of an exciting new life in an exciting new land, and in September 1957 I joined the world-famous clinic – though not as a practicing clinician. As had happened twice before in planning my career, I had changed my mind about which professional path to follow. Neither a career in civil engineering nor with the church suited me, although the latter might have seemed preordained for me given the family I was born into.

early years

The road to Mayo for me began in the small town of Portglenone in Northern Ireland. I was born in the evening on May 21, 1919, in the front bedroom of the village's Presbyterian parsonage, where my father, the Reverend William Frederick Shepherd, and my mother, Matilda (Tilly) Thompson Shepherd, lived. The manse's ample grounds included a tennis court, a soccer field, and a driveway constructed of sharp stones. My brothers and I—Harry was four years my senior and Fred, two—often raced one another around the driveway on our bicycles, suffering inevitable cuts and bruises.

Family life centered on our father's typical duties as a clergyman, which included calling on the aged and sick of his congregation in their homes. He often recounted the time he visited an elderly woman for whom cleanliness was not much of a virtue. After a prayer she served tea, and my father noticed that one side of the cup was dirty. As a precaution, he held the cup in his left hand and drank from its clean side. When he had nearly finished, the woman said, "Ah, Minister! I see that you are left-handed like myself."

Unable to afford any other mode of conveyance, Father made his rounds on a bicycle—a physical challenge in the steep hills of Portglenone, since bicycles back then had no adjustable gears. Some members of his congregation eventually bought him a secondhand motorcycle, which made his rounds easier. Since the motorcycle had a sidecar, my mother often accompanied him on his visits. My brother Harry and I learned to drive the old motorcycle, and, without Father guiding us from the sidecar, we would prowl the local roads early in the morning—before the police came around, that is.

Father's duties also included entertaining prominent members of the congregation. Our usual custom was to have a buffet dinner at the parsonage followed by a sing-along, with my mother—a capable pianist—as the accompanist.

With Harry and Fred, I attended a Protestant school for boys across the road from our father's church. The obnoxious headmaster dealt with offenses, including the failure to learn, by beating the offender's hand, palm up, with a bamboo cane. Once, when the headmaster was beating a boy, a friend of the unfortunate offender—the school bully—seized the master's cane and hit him vigorously on the back of his head and his bottom as the master rushed for the door. Both the headmaster and the bully were dismissed from the school as a consequence. My parents decided my brothers and I should get our education elsewhere.

Soon thereafter my father saw a better opportunity in Raphoe in County

Donegal in Ireland. Like the Presbyterian manse we moved from, the one in Raphoe was a large house with considerable grounds for a tennis court and a vegetable garden. We boys grew up living off the abundance of the garden; the vegetables, tomatoes, raspberries, and strawberries were fresh for every meal. Mother began brewing her own alcohol, an unlikely activity that we kept secret from the parishioners. Unlike drinking, however, dancing was permissible. We often invited younger members of the congregation to join us in a loft above an outbuilding that housed Father's motorcycle; there, we danced to the tunes of gramophone records.

Mother first made home-brewed alcohol during her early experiences on the farm where she grew up, not far from the parsonage where I was born. She and her two younger sisters were raised by their three unmarried uncles. The girls' mother had left them to seek the solace of another man after their father died, the rumor being that she had cavorted with a Presbyterian minister in a different parish and that he had been dismissed from the church. Neither my brothers nor I ever heard the name of our maternal grandmother mentioned by our mother or aunts.

Father's family history was decidedly more conventional. After graduating from divinity school in Belfast, he traveled to the United States, where he earned a bachelor's degree in divinity at Princeton Theological Seminary and became an assistant minister in a church in New Jersey. About this same time, his older brother, Harry, persuaded their father—my paternal grandfather, who was a Presbyterian minister in Ballyrooney, Northern Ireland—to accompany him across the Atlantic. Harry was engaged to a young woman he had met a few years earlier, and he wanted his father to perform the marriage ceremony in New York. After the wedding in 1908 in a church in Brooklyn, my grandfather exercised the parental authority characteristic of the times to persuade my father, then twenty-eight, to return with him to Ireland a few weeks later. According to family myth, my grandfather convinced Father that the pension plan for ministers was better in Northern Ireland than in America!

Uncle Harry had met his bride, Velma Tyler, during the several years he lived in Canada and the United States. Her parents lived in Ontario, but she was then in nurse's training in a New York hospital. Their courtship continued by correspondence after Harry returned to Northern Ireland and entered the medical school of Queen's University in Belfast. He graduated in 1906 as one of the top six students in a class of eighty-five, but home held little attraction for the new doctor. "Practicing medicine in Ireland is out of the question," he wrote Velma, "as it is overstocked with doctors."

Harry responded to an advertisement in the *British Medical Journal,* placed by an aging physician for an assistant in his general medical practice in the center of a large coal-mining district in England. After he was hired, Harry moved in 1906 to South Shields, a busy shipbuilding seaport near Newcastle-on-Tyne. In the custom of his time, Harry visited his patients in their homes, using a bicycle or occasionally a horse and trap.

"My chief, the old man, is a miser, stingy as the devil in every way," he wrote Velma. Yet he was able to accumulate a little money, and thus persuade Velma to marry him. The newlyweds sailed for England and settled in South Shields, where their only child, Eleanor, was born in 1913. The same year he became a father, Harry joined the Fourth Northumbrian Howitzer Brigade with the rank of lieutenant. The following year, Harry died unexpectedly at his home at age thirty-eight, probably of a heart attack. Though he had practiced medicine in South Shields only six years, he was respected throughout the community, and he received a full military funeral. A riderless horse, stirrups reversed, followed his coffin.

Velma took Eleanor back to Canada and took up social work in Toronto. She remarried in 1923, to William Leask, who also died suddenly, at age forty-five. Eleanor qualified as a nurse and married William Cameron. They had three sons: Donald, now living in Sydney, Australia; David, who died at the age of twenty-two; and William, now living in Toronto.

Harry's sudden death at such a young age was notable in my long-lived family. His sister, my Aunt Lena, lived to be ninety-nine, and his brother, my father, until he was eighty-five. My father died in June 1970, five years after the death of my mother in August 1965 at age seventy-three.

Aunt Lena, who was six years younger than my father, was my favorite aunt, in part because she was so direct. I remember she described a man who courted her years earlier as "the sort of man who sits down to pee." After she earned a bachelor's degree from Trinity College in Dublin, she married a Presbyterian minister, William Morrow. They moved to Bangor, a seaside town in Northern Ireland, where she became the major caregiver to Grandmother and Grandfather Shepherd. A few years after her marriage, Lena's husband had a brain hemorrhage and became paralyzed, so she nursed him too until he died of a second hemorrhage. Thus, long before World War II, Aunt Lena's husband, parents, and brother Harry were dead.

Lena was head of the Red Cross in Bangor during the war and afterward married James Cunningham, a widower. She had been long-time friends of both Cunninghams. James had worked until retirement in a government office in Belfast, and after they married, they managed his farm in County Derry in Northern Ireland. James soon developed vascular disease. By then, I was researching vascular disease in the physiology department at Queen's University in Belfast and Aunt Lena asked me to examine her husband. The blood flow to his legs showed that the disease was advanced, and he died about five years after their marriage. She returned to Bangor, where she continued her work with the Red Cross until her death.

Robert Kirk, a relative of my paternal grandmother, was the only family member with money. He sold expensive automobiles in Northern Ireland and owned a tile factory in England. The Kirks lived in a mansion called "The Pines" a few miles outside Belfast. In earlier years my grandparents visited them frequently, and Aunt Lena was a close friend of Robert Kirk's daughter, Eileen. Eileen's brother, Allister, was uninterested in his father's business, preferring the social life instead. Allister sometimes visited us unexpectedly at the parsonage in Portglenone. He always arrived in a supercharged, expensive sports car, often on a Sunday afternoon, his breath usually smelling of alcohol. Staunch Presbyterians in those days regarded alcohol as an invention of the devil, so my parents always hoped we would have no other visitors on these occasions! Those were years when wealthy people sent such children to Australia, paying them a remittance as long as they lived overseas. Thus, Allister became a remittance man in Sydney.

Campbell College

Though the salary paid my father in Raphoe was small, it was somewhat higher than what he had received from his old congregation in Portglenone, enough so that he could help to educate his three sons.

In his youth, my father had attended a private male preparatory school in Belfast City, the capital of Northern Ireland. The school was named Campbell College for the farmer who had donated the land and given the money to build it. In his will, Campbell stipulated that the sons of Presbyterian ministers could attend without paying tuition. Most of the students were boarders, including my brothers and me. To ensure that the students from rich and less rich families could not be distinguished by their dress, all boys wore the same uniform: black jacket, white shirt, school tie, gray trousers, and black shoes.

At nine-and-a-half, however, I was too young to enter the main school with Harry and Fred, so I went first to Cabin Hill, a primary school near

Campbell College. A country house, formerly the home of a nobleman, Cabin Hill had opened the same year I entered. Tennyson's famous line of Ulysses exhorting his men to embark with him on a final voyage became the motto of Cabin Hill: "To strive, to seek, to find, and not to yield."

All meals were served in the refectory. On the philosophy that it is sinful to waste food, Cabin Hill required students to eat all the food served them. One boy who sat beside me could not abide the nearly cold porridge and put his serving in a handkerchief to dispose of after breakfast each day. At first he got rid of it under a bush behind the school, but when the bush succumbed after about a year, he had to find a new location. He continued this routine every single day of his three years at the school!

Each evening at bedtime we had to attend a brief religious service, which included singing a hymn. From time to time the headmaster's aunt crossed the Irish Sea by ferry to visit him at the school. We always knew when she was in transit because the headmaster, C. B. Lace, would select the hymn "O Hear Us When We Cry to Thee for Those in Peril on the Sea." Once, when she was late, we kept singing it over and over until she appeared. She took her dinner with us each night in the dining room, usually finishing before we did. She would then rise from the table and slowly ascend the staircase to her room. She was a buxom woman, and her large rear end wobbled with each step she took. We called her "Ma Bumwobbler."

One day we received a visit from a prominent Irish poet, who charged each of us to write a poem. My oldest brother, Harry, encouraged me to write one about the famous yearly Tourist Trophy road race for cars in Northern Ireland, which our family always attended. Stimulated by memories of what had happened in the race the previous year (1930), I wrote:

When we were last at Bradshaw's Bray,
'Twas on the Tourist Trophy day.
We saw throughout the opera lens
The speed of the Mercedes-Benz.
But the Bentley came much faster.
Speeding round, it went on past her,
Until they reached the eighteenth lap.
The Bentley, leading, got a clap.
Just then the rains began to fall.
The roads got very wet.
The Bentley, skidding, went into a wall
And hasn't been mended yet.

Auto-racing historians may recall that 1930 was also the year that Bentley won the Le Mans twenty-four-hour endurance race for the fifth time, overtaking a Mercedes at 130 miles an hour. Bentley, however, has not reentered since. Remarkably enough, I won the competition, and my poem was published in the school magazine—my first and only effort at poetry.

Having been caned on the hand at my first school in Portglenone, I soon found that the punishment for offenses at Cabin Hill and Campbell College was a beating on the bottom with a bamboo cane. This happened to me on two occasions at Cabin Hill. The first time was when I arrived late to class one morning, eating a banana my mother had sent. The other time was on my last night at Cabin Hill, when on a dare I leaped from a tall cupboard onto my bed, whose metal springs gave way. The springs, the mattress, and I landed on the floor. It was impossible to repair the bed, but I disguised the problem by anchoring myself under the bedclothes while the master turned out the lights. After he left I retrieved the mattress, spread it on the floor, and lay there to sleep. But some of my classmates created a disturbance, and the master returned. When he switched on the lights, it was plain my bed was empty. He called my name and led me to the headmaster, who administered six strokes to my bottom.

Having reached age thirteen, I was ready to go on to Campbell College. At the final recognition ceremony at Cabin Hill, the headmaster recited "A Psalm of Life" by Henry Wadsworth Longfellow, one of my favorite poems:

Lives of great men all remind us
We can make our lives sublime,
And, departing, leave behind us
Footprints on the sands of time.

The headmaster followed this by saying that I had indeed left my footprints!

Campbell College had all the traditions of the English public schools (the equivalent of private schools in the United States), and I quickly learned my standing there. Harry, my oldest brother, was addressed formally as "Shepherd Major" and Fred, the next brother, as "Shepherd Minor." I was "Shepherd Minimus," a moniker that sorely tested my self-esteem. Circumstances improved after my brothers departed for medical school and I became head prefect. As such, I was charged with disciplining students who infringed on school rules by administering a bamboo cane to their bottoms. Having held the school record for being caned previous to my new responsibilities, however, I seldom exercised this privilege.

When a teacher decreed punishment and announced the number of strokes (usually four), a student had the right of appeal to the headmaster. The prevailing opinion among students, however, was that any appeal meant the headmaster would automatically increase the number of strokes to the maximum of six. Before delivering a caning, the teachers would pat your bottom to check that you had not inserted padding. (I had heard that horsehair properly inserted would break the cane, but my first experience in research disproved this.)

Many churches had both noon and 6:00 P.M. services on Sundays. At Campbell College, we dressed for church in black suits with white shirts (the school colors) with hard collars, bow ties, and straw hats. We walked in line to the local Episcopalian or Presbyterian church for both services and all sat together. The school prefects passed collection plates at the appropriate time, while we challenged one another to *pretend* to contribute without being detected.

The great English composer Ralph Vaughan Williams once visited Campbell College and conducted the school choir, reminding the singers that "the only correct music is that which is beautiful and noble." That was a reach for me. For some reason I was a member of the choir, even though I cannot sing. In those days of the British empire, especially on important national anniversaries, we sang "Coronation Ode" to the melody "Pomp and Circumstance," from Edward Elgar's 1902 *Land of Hope and Glory:*

> *Land of Hope and Glory,*
> *Mother of the Free,*
> *How shall we extol thee,*
> *Who are born of thee?*
> *Wider still and wider*
> *Shall thy bounds be set;*
> *God, who made thee mighty,*
> *Make thee mightier yet.*

On appropriate occasions, we also sang the school anthem, whose chorus exclaimed, "Campbell, Campbell, Campbell, the school that we love so well." Singing sotto voce, some students substituted a different line in the chorus: "Campbell, Campbell, Campbell, the school that we hate like hell."

The only scholastic prize I won at Campbell College was a book, *Scott's Journey to the Pole.* I should mention that the prize was awarded in a religion class that I shared with two other uninterested students. I did, however, excel at athletics and at age seventeen became the first student from Campbell College to participate in the Public Schools Athletic Competition at the White City Stadium in London. I won the half-mile race in the semifinals but came in third the next day in the finals. A national newspaper reporter wrote that "Shepherd ran without confidence," and I suspect he was right.

(Much later, I had the good fortune to meet Roger Bannister, the first person to run the mile in less than four minutes—3:59.4 at Oxford University on May 6, 1954—for which he was knighted. When I knew him, Sir Roger was a consultant neurologist in the British National Health Service, and we had similar interests in the regulation of arterial blood pressure in humans. For the 1999 edition of his classic book, *A Textbook of Clinical Disorders of the Autonomic Nervous System,* coedited with Christopher Mathias, Bannister invited me and my son, Roger, now a Mayo Clinic internist specializing in cardiovascular disease, to contribute the chapter "Control of Blood Pressure and the Circulation in Man.")

After Campbell College, my brothers decided on medicine as a career, and both Harry and Fred entered the medical school of Queen's University in Belfast. There was some thought in the family that I might follow my father and grandfather into the ministry, and I began to study Latin and Greek, prerequisites for entrance into Presbyterian College, a theological institution. Before I graduated from Campbell, however, my family recognized, as did I, that I should think of a more suitable career.

During the period after high school when I was wondering what to do, Aunt Lena asked our wealthy distant relative Robert Kirk for suggestions. Kirk offered to hire me to develop suitable colors for the tiles his firm manufactured in England. By chance, one of my friends, also the son of a Presbyterian minister, worked at the tile factory. When I visited him, he advised me not to accept what he described as a dead-end job. I agreed with his assessment, and my career took another course.

after Campbell College

My headmaster at Campbell, who had been a colonel in a British regiment during World War I, suggested that I seek a job with a local railway. His friend and former army colleague, the chief executive officer of the railway, hired me to apprentice with the civil engineering group. He said eventually I might pass the many requirements and qualify as a civil engineer.

My initial assignment was to make detailed drawings of portions of the railway track broken by the trains, but I also had the opportunity to make a genuine public contribution. Years earlier, the railway had acquired land in a beautiful glen leading down to the sea. This land became a favorite public park, and the railway had decided it should provide toilet facilities for the park's many visitors. I was to design these facilities, with the instruction that I should do only the minimum necessary. I selected the space, secured the necessary urinals, and supervised the construction of roof and walls. Years later, after my appointment to the staff of the Mayo Clinic, my family and I revisited Ireland. When I showed them my handiwork at the park, they immediately christened the toilets "John's johns"!

When I began work at the railroad in the late 1930s, the wooden joists that once spanned rock buttresses supporting the railway tracks over small streams were being replaced with concrete joists reinforced by steel rods. When a new set of joists was ready, a work crew took it to the site. As soon as the day's last train had passed, the men lifted the track, removed the wooden joists, put the concrete ones in position, and replaced the track in time for the first train the next morning. After I had worked in the engineering office for some time, a colleague asked me to help him design such a set of concrete replacement joists. The joists we designed were duly made and delivered to the site. But after the workmen removed the wooden joists, they discovered that the concrete ones were too short to span the buttresses! You can imagine the panic they felt as they labored to restore the old joists in time for the morning train. To this day, I am baffled as to who made the incorrect measurements.

By this time I had concluded that engineering did not inspire me. At age nineteen, I decided my path led toward medicine.

medical school

In my final year at Campbell, I took and passed the matriculation examination for London University. At the time, I had no thought of medicine, but my record helped me earn admission in 1939 to Queen's University in Belfast. During my first year at the university I had to concentrate on science courses, since my studies in Latin and Greek at Campbell had reduced the time I spent studying those subjects. Before I could obtain approval to transfer to the medical school, I had to pass courses in chemistry, physics, botany, and zoology. Another student, a woman, also was admitted under these conditions, while other members of our class were taking the regular courses of the medical school. Both of us passed with distinction, and I am still grateful to the dean and faculty of the medical school who approved our transfer.

They said we were qualified to make up the missed courses and eligible to graduate in the usual time of six years. In the British Isles, students can enter medical school directly from high school, without additional time in a liberal arts college.

Aunt Lena and my mother, with money she received from the sale of her family farm, agreed to pay my tuition. A fellow student and I once decided to help out with the cost of medical school by breeding and selling pedigreed bull terrier dogs. Bull terriers were developed in England as a cross between bulldogs and a now extinct breed of terrier. We bought a young bull terrier named Pip of Spunkane and a female. Pip was affectionate, but the female turned out to be vicious, even to her owners. The veterinarian we consulted said that she was not only incurable, but that we were in danger of being sued for her behavior. We had to have her—and our moneymaking scheme—put down. I gave Pip to my mother as a replacement for her Irish terrier that had just died, and they enjoyed several years together.

My class, which was typical of medical schools in the British Isles, was about two-thirds men and one-third women. As far as I could observe, the women were treated in all respects the same as the men. In my anatomy class, in fact, it was evident that some of the two genders collaborated in learning the anatomical complexities of the reproductive organs.

When we students met in the theater before each lecture, we often broke into song before the lecturer arrived. These were not classic songs, but those made up by the vocalists who led us, without regard to conventional behavior. I recall one such song, whose lyrics went: "Oh, the eagles they fly high in Moville / The eagles they fly high, and they shit right in your eye. / Aren't you glad the cows don't fly in Moville!" We wisely stopped singing in time to cheer the arrival of the lecturer.

A memorable incident during medical school took place during one of my clinical rotations at the Fever Hospital a few miles from Belfast. In those days, when infectious diseases were common, many patients entered specialty hospitals for treatment. On one occasion, the chief resident said that he wished to advise us medical students and that we should assemble on a lawn outside the hospital. The five of us (all men) obeyed. The chief resident then reappeared with a shotgun, lined us up in single file, and said he was teaching a lesson in obedience. When he yelled "Jump!" we had better obey him, for he was going to fire at the ground where our feet had been. He was obviously drunk, but we obeyed his commands faithfully. When he paused to reload, we rushed to disarm him.

the Second World War

When Germany invaded Poland in September 1939, Britain and France declared war on Germany. As medical students, my classmates and I became part of a "reserved occupation." This meant we could not join the armed forces until after graduation. Maintaining the output of doctors was more important than signing up more recruits. Instead, we joined the Home Guard, a volunteer force trained to protect the homeland against the Germans. An invasion seemed inevitable after the fall of France and the subsequent rescue of the British Expeditionary Force at Dunkirk. I awaited the coming of the Germans across the English Channel in that cloudless summer of 1940 while clinging to my World War I–vintage rifle and ten rounds of ammunition.

As members of the Home Guard, we put on our uniforms for training in battle tactics after medical school lectures. The Battle of Britain had begun, waged in the air by the Royal Air Force and Hermann Göring's feared Luftwaffe. Day after day the Germans came, and day after day the valiant RAF fighter pilots rose to oppose them.

At first, we had taken up our Home Guard duties at watch posts along the coast, but our assignment changed as the threat of invasion began to fade and we endured daily air bombardment. My home city of Belfast, with its large shipyards, including that of Harlan and Wolff (where the ill-fated luxury liner *Titanic* was built thirty years earlier), was now busy constructing battleships. It was an obvious target for the German bombers. Their nightly forays missed the shipyards, however, and instead destroyed large sections of the city. With many of my fellow medical students, I stood with binoculars on the roof of the main teaching hospital as the German planes dropped their bombs. Our purpose was to spot where the bombs fell and help rescue the injured from the wreckage. We quickly learned that as soon as they dropped their bombs, the bombers flew low over the city and strafed the streets with their machine guns. One of my colleagues was killed just this way. Even today, you can see pockmarks from German bullets on many of Belfast's buildings, silent testimony of these events more than sixty years ago.

The losses were terrible that summer, but slowly the tide turned. Finally, on August 20, 1940, in an address before the House of Commons, Winston Churchill declared victory in the Battle of Britain. In 1940 and throughout most of 1941, the British Commonwealth stood almost alone against Germany and the other Axis powers, but we felt reassured by President Franklin Roosevelt's Lend Lease program, under which the United States provided merchant ships to Britain. As part of the arrangement, American frigates helped escort the battered convoys of merchant ships through mine-studded and submarine-infested seas to deliver essential supplies to Britain.

British crews came to the United States and helped man these frigates. My brother Fred was then in service as a surgeon-lieutenant in the British navy. In early 1942, he and some 120 British sailors manned an American frigate in Providence, Rhode Island, and took it to Boston, then to New York, where they joined a convoy for England. Later, he served on a battleship that supported the Allied landings in Italy at the Battle of Salerno. After the war ended in 1945, those who had been the first to join the armed forces were the first out. As the time of Fred's discharge approached, however, he was unexpectedly assigned to duty in Australia. He informed the admiralty that the date of his discharge would occur before he had completed the long sea voyage to Sydney. Bureaucracy being what it is, he still had to go. As soon as he arrived in Sydney, Fred informed the authorities that his time was up—and they sent him back at once to Northern Ireland by air!

My oldest brother, Harry, had joined the Royal Air Force in 1940 after medical school. He became a squadron leader assigned first to an antisubmarine unit of Sunderland flying boats operating off the west coast of Africa in the British Gold Coast (now Ghana), then to an RAF hospital in Takoradi, also on the Gold Coast. After the North African campaign, Harry served as a radiologist at an RAF hospital at Holton, near London, then at a hospital in Yorkshire. After the war, he returned to civilian life and the Royal Victoria Hospital in Belfast, then to the Radcliffe Infirmary in Oxford, England. At Radcliffe, he trained in neuroradiology under the distinguished neurosurgeon Sir Hugh Cairns. Harry returned to Belfast after receiving an appointment to the staff of the Royal Victoria Hospital as a consultant in neuroradiology.

marriage

World War II was nearly over by the time I graduated from medical school at Queen's University in 1945. I had earned the three customary degrees: an M.B. (bachelor of medicine), a B.Ch. (bachelor of surgery), and a B.A.O. (bachelor of the arts of obstetrics). With the end of the war, the military no longer needed so many doctors, and so I did not serve in the armed forces. I decided to begin postgraduate training at the Royal Victoria Hospital, the main university teaching hospital in Belfast, as an assistant to the professor and chair of surgery at my medical school at Queen's University.

Typical of the ranking order in the European medical community, his word was law and his subordinates were never to question his decisions. On one such occasion he stated that anyone who wished to succeed should keep his mouth closed and his bowels open. One day after performing a surgery, his ego was bruised when he emerged from the shower just as a female nurse entered the staff dressing room by mistake. "Shepherd, would you believe it?" he said to me after dressing. "She never even *looked* at me!"

(Some years later a similar incident involved the son of Charles Mayo, one of the two famous Mayo brothers. One evening Chuck Mayo was alone in the surgeon's lounge after a long day of operating. One of the Sisters of Saint Francis came in to tidy up the lounge just as he stepped from the shower without benefit of cover. The nun stared at him in astonishment, and he at her. Then he looked her in the eye and said, "From now on call me Chuck!")

My professor suggested that I too become a surgeon—but if I chose to follow his advice, I should avoid involvement with the opposite sex. In his customary straightforward terms, and in the masculine behavior of the time, he counseled me to consider what a woman looks like at 3:00 A.M. sitting on a chamber pot with her hair down. He told me that to succeed during the long training program to become a surgeon, I should keep my balls in ice for the next five years.

His warnings came too late. I had met my fiancé, Helen Mary Johnston, in July 1944 in Portnoo in County Donegal. Our family vacationed in Portnoo each August, and I had arrived early with a colleague to study for my final medical examinations. Helen, a secretary to the manager of a company in Belfast, was also on vacation in Portnoo with her mother and father, who headed a Belfast import/export business. I first saw Helen as she strolled with her parents past a pier for small lobster boats toward a path favored by tourists for its spectacular view of islands and headlands.

That summer I had grown my first (and only) beard. When I saw this attractive young woman I decided to shave it off, leaving only my mustache. The following day I sat alone in my swimsuit on the pier, planning, when I saw her again, to dive into the sea from the top of the twenty-foot wall at the end of the pier, hoping this might impress her. When she and her parents did appear, I dived into the sea, and they walked down the pier to watch me. Thus we talked, and her parents invited me to join them the next day for a long car tour of other beautiful places in County Donegal.

This opportunity allowed me to walk and talk together with Helen, and our relationship progressed rapidly. We married a year later, on July 28, 1945, in the Rosemary Presbyterian Church, which she attended, in Belfast. My father conducted the marriage ceremony. My cousin, David Irwin, was my best man; he too was in his final year of medical school at Trinity College in Dublin. The professor who had advised me to choose surgery over marriage attended our wedding, along with his wife. Helen and I honeymooned in a delightful place with an outstanding hotel, Rosapenna, on the seaside in the northern part of County Donegal.

My year-long term at Royal Victoria Hospital ended in June 1946. My further training, scheduled with Professor Henry Barcroft in the Department of Physiology at Queen's University, would not begin until October. To earn money during the three-month interval, with a little time spent vacationing with Helen and my family at Portnoo that August, I became an assistant to a general medical practitioner in the newly organized British National Health Service.

His practice was conducted in a large three-story house in Belfast. The waiting rooms for patients were on the ground floor. The physician's office was on the first floor, and at the top of the stairs leading to this floor was a landing with a table laden with government forms for patients. My instructions were to stand at this table as the secretary at the bottom of the stairs announced the name of the patient assigned to me. As the patient ascended the stairs, I was to determine the problem and have the appropriate form ready as the patient came to my table. I was to examine the patient only as a last resort. In this way, I could see many patients in quick succession, sometimes thirty or forty during a single evening. Since the money paid to the physician depended on the number of patients seen, this approach certainly enhanced his income.

When the physician was in his office in the evenings, his secretary was to send only certain female patients to him. When he left for vacation, his only instructions to the secretary were to have the examination table in his office fixed because it creaked! Wisely, I did not quote to him Hippocrates' advice to physicians, the wisdom of keeping himself "far from all intentional ill-doing and seduction, and especially from the pleasures of love with women."

I had taken the job at the suggestion of a colleague who preceded me as the physician's assistant. Despite his advice—"Why worry? It's good money"—I could not wait to complete the job. In retrospect, I can see that this treadmill approach to patient care may have forecast the changes in American medicine. Of for-profit health maintenance organizations, or HMOs, it has been said that *caveat aeger* (let the patient beware) has replaced *caveat emptor* (let the buyer beware).

learning about Mayo

In August 1946, the summer before my postgraduate studies began with Professor Barcroft, my family reunited after years of war at our annual vacation site in County Donegal, on the northwest coast of Ireland. What a change! Gone were the tall vertical wooden poles driven deeply at close intervals in the sandy beaches to deter German planes from landing with invading troops. Gone too were the bodies of sailors washed ashore from merchant ships sunk off the Irish coast by German submarines.

During that happy, peaceful month, my brother Fred gave me a book that changed my life. One day during the war, while waiting for an American frigate to join the merchant ship convoy to England, Fred had gone into a medical bookstore in Boston. Some American physicians who happened to be in the store at the same time enthusiastically recommended *The Doctors Mayo.*

As I sat reading the book on an Irish headland looking westward over the Atlantic toward North America, I became fascinated by Helen Clapesattle's 1941 story of William Worrall Mayo, father of the famous Mayo brothers, William James and Charles Horace. W. W. Mayo was born in the English village of Eccles, a few miles from Manchester. Succumbing to a strong vision of America, he sailed for New York in 1845 at the age of twenty-five.

During the Civil War, W. W. Mayo was appointed examining surgeon of the army enrollment board for the First Minnesota District, which included the southern half of the state. The board's headquarters were in the small town of Rochester, connected by railroad in 1864 to the Mississippi River port of Winona. The Union army required all men to register for military service: anyone wishing exemption from the draft had the right to appear before the enrollment board. Many such cases involved claims of physical disability, of course, and this set in motion a trek of the sick to Rochester to be examined by Dr. Mayo.

The Union army may have decided the future site of the Mayo Clinic, but it was a devastating tornado that launched Saint Marys Hospital. So many people were injured in the twister that struck Rochester on August 21, 1883, that Mother Mary Alfred Moes of the Sisters of Saint Francis was convinced that a hospital was needed. She volunteered the nuns to earn money for the hospital's construction, provided Mayo and his sons, Dr. Will and Dr. Charlie, would be the physicians.

Clapesattle traced in her book how the Mayo Clinic developed under the leadership of the Mayo brothers. They were skilled surgeons who established the group practice of medicine, despite suspicions and opposition in an era of individual practitioners. Though at the top of their profession, each brother visited medical centers around the world to gain knowledge and add it to their surgical practice. The author wrote that Dr. Will "could say he had studied surgery in every town in America and Canada of one hundred thousand population or more, and had crossed the Atlantic thirty times—not to mention the side trips to Alaska, Cuba, the Antipodes, and South America. And Dr. Charlie was not much less traveled." I was pleased to note that Dr. Charlie received an honorary degree in 1925 from my alma mater, Queen's University of Belfast.

Decades later, Dr. Charlie's son told several wonderful anecdotes about his famous ancestors in his 1968 book *Mayo: The Story of My Family and My Career: The Autobiography of Dr. Charles ("Chuck") Mayo.* One such story addressed why a world-famous medical facility should have located in Minnesota: "I have a feeling that the main reason Grandfather allowed his family to root in Rochester was that Grandmother finally put her foot down and told him she would wander no more." Another story told of W. W. Mayo at age ninety getting his hand stuck in a corn-shucking machine, which caught and crushed his fingers. "Anyone who knows as much about farming as W. W.," sniffed his son Will, "should have better sense than to stick his hand in a shucker." The old doctor exploded and ordered him from the room. "Only Charlie will take care of me!" he shouted.

Even my brother Fred was able to recount a story involving the Mayo brothers that he had heard during his time at the naval barracks in Boston. During the war, the United States developed a crash program to mass-produce Liberty ships, small merchant cargo ships with a maximum speed of eleven knots. The "Libs," as they were nicknamed, played an important role in supplying American troops overseas. In December 1942, still early in the program, the Delta Shipbuilding Company of New Orleans launched the Liberty ship *S.S. Mayo Brothers.* The honor of christening her by breaking a bottle of champagne across her bow went to Cecile Carlson, a Minnesota high school student who became the state's champion scrap-metal collector after persuading her uncle to donate an outdated thirteen-ton tractor! (After the war ended, a number of Liberty ships—the *S.S. Mayo Brothers* among them—ended up in the National Defense Reserve Fleet at Mobile, Alabama, then as scrap a few years later. Thus did the *S.S. Mayo Brothers,* by then renamed No. 242674, return to scrap as it had begun.)

The Doctors Mayo thoroughly captured my imagination, and I knew that one day I must witness this medical miracle firsthand.

postgraduate medical training

After my summer with the British National Health Service, I was glad to begin the academic year in October 1946. To qualify as a surgeon, I had to fulfill the requirements to become a fellow of one of the Royal College of Surgeons—of England, Ireland, or Scotland. The examinations for each college were similar and consisted of two parts: the first covered the basic medical sciences; the second, years of surgical training followed by the final clinical examinations. To pass the first part I followed the custom of taking a year from clinical responsibilities to spend in a basic science department in the medical school, and thus soak up the knowledge necessary to pass the exam. Since earlier I had enjoyed Professor Henry Barcroft's lectures, I selected the Department of Physiology at Queen's University. Barcroft was completely unselfish, always giving the young people who worked with him every opportunity to develop their talents. He offered me a modest stipend for assisting students in the practical classes.

Barcroft came from a distinguished Irish Quaker family. His grandfather, also named Henry Barcroft, invented the Bessbrook weaving machine in 1869. His mother was a daughter of Sir Robert Ball, who was Astronomer Royal of Ireland before becoming Lowndean Professor of Astronomy and Geometry at Cambridge University. His father, Joseph Barcroft, was internationally known for his classic studies on physiological function; he was appointed chair of physiology at Cambridge University in 1925 and knighted.

Henry Barcroft married Bridget Mary (Biddy) Ramsey in 1935. The eldest daughter of A. S. Ramsey, president of Magdalene College at Cambridge, she had just graduated from the London School of Medicine for Women. That same year, Barcroft was appointed to the Dunville Chair of Physiology at Queen's University, then the fourth largest medical school in the British Isles. He was thirty years old. The school had a reputation for sound clinical instruction but not for research. The university's expectation was that Barcroft would stimulate research within the medical school, which he did.

Barcroft was the first to demonstrate the effect of sympathetic nerves on human blood vessels. When activated, these nerves cause the blood vessels to constrict. Based on Barcroft's studies, surgeons during World War II operated to remove these nerves to the limb blood vessels as they emerged from the spinal column in soldiers whose limb arteries had to be tied off after gunshot wounds. The point was to increase the blood supply to the limb by opening bypass vessels around the ligated main arteries, thus avoiding the necessity for amputation. Barcroft, of course, knew that I was a budding surgeon, and he challenged me to determine whether this assumption was correct. He suggested that I measure the blood flow to one leg in young healthy subjects during temporary occlusion of the femoral artery to that leg, before and after blocking the sympathetic nerves. The object was to see if these vessels were under nervous control.

Barcroft informed me that a thesis of my study could lead to a master of surgery degree, which would further my plans for a surgical career. (This was later facilitated by the award in 1949 of a British Medical Association scholarship.) I did indeed demonstrate the importance of these nerves, and the English surgeon whom Barcroft selected to examine my thesis was a great advocate of dividing these nerves in patients with circulatory problems. To my delight, he recommended that I receive a gold medal with my master's degree in 1948. Because gold was scarce at the time, however, the citation was honorary. (I did not receive the medal until 1977—and then only in silver gilt rather than gold due to inflation. Ian Roddie, an earlier associate who had become dean of Queen's University medical school, invited my son, Roger, then a medical student at Queen's, to accept the medal on my behalf. Later, I won the Williamson Prize, given by the Queen's University medical faculty for the "most distinguished published work by a graduate of not more than ten years standing.")

a career as a medical scientist

I enjoyed my research experience, and when Barcroft offered me a tenured position as a lecturer in the physiology department, I changed my career focus. I gave up the idea of becoming a surgeon in favor of a career as a medical scientist.

From 1948 until 1953, I conducted research and lectured at Queen's. One of my responsibilities was to give formal morning lectures in physiology to medical students in their preclinical years. Queen's offered two places for qualified students from America entering the medical school. One such student, who was from New York City and some years older than the others, soon informed me that he did not like rising in time for my 9:00 A.M. lectures. He proposed that a fellow student place a tape recorder on the podium where I talked, and he would retrieve this later. I carefully explained to him that in our backward system the attendance of each student was compulsory.

Later, this same student took a novel approach to making money in Ireland as he pursued his medical studies. After learning that contraceptives were illegal in Eire and that there was no duty on cameras purchased there (the duty was high on such equipment in Northern Ireland), he smuggled condoms by car into Dublin and on the return trip smuggled cameras into Belfast. When word of his activities reached the customs agents who checked traffic across the border between Eire and Northern Ireland, the student was caught, accused of smuggling, and summoned to appear in court. He came to tell me he had made a boodle—and to ask how much would it cost to settle with the judge! I first explained that attempting a bribe would not be a good idea, and then I advised him to submit his resignation at once to the university, since I knew he would be expelled automatically if he were convicted and sentenced by the court. This would be on his record, to the detriment of applications he might make to other schools. He resigned, was found guilty, and fined. He left Belfast, and I never heard of him again.

In 1950, Henry Barcroft accepted the position of professor of physiology at St. Thomas's Hospital Medical School in London. His successor was David Greenfield, who came from St. Mary's Medical School, also in London. This was an exciting time, since I was able to continue my research on the human cardiovascular system. My colleagues and I had demonstrated the importance of signals coming to the brain from the heart and lungs that regulated the arterial blood pressure. Consequently, I received the M.D. degree with gold medal in 1951. This degree illustrates one of the differences between medical education in the United Kingdom and the United States: in the U.K., an M.D. is a higher-level degree, while in the United States it is the entry degree.

With my colleagues, I regularly visited London to present research papers at meetings of the Physiological Society. On such visits, we stayed at large, relatively inexpensive hotels. Guests often left their shoes outside their hotel room doors at night, which the hotel staff would then collect, polish, and return early in the morning. My prankish friends and I occasionally succumbed to the temptation to redistribute the shoes to different doors, which caused some interesting responses by the guests involved.

to the United States

By the 1950s long catheters could be passed safely from veins in the arms into the chambers of the heart and into the arteries leading to the lungs. This opened the possibility for increased knowledge of the normal functioning of the heart and of changes due to congenital and acquired heart disease. At that time, catheters were being used in this way at three leading medical centers: one in London, one in New York City, and one in Rochester, Minnesota, that place I had read about in *The Doctors Mayo.*

Heart disease interested me as an area of research, and I realized I could enhance my career if I conducted studies at another important academic center besides Queen's University. Might I do such work at Mayo Clinic? I knew that Jeremy Swan, a former colleague and fellow Irishman, had joined Mayo after earning a doctorate for his research under the tutelage of Henry Barcroft, my mentor. Since I was due a sabbatical year at Queen's University, I wrote to Jeremy about the possibility of a position. Through his influence, I received an invitation to be research assistant at the Mayo Clinic in the physiology section, which I enthusiastically accepted. I would work with Jeremy Swan and Earl Wood, both acknowledged leaders in the application of this new technique of cardiac catheterization.

Even before my connection to Mayo came about through Swan and Barcroft, even before I had read *The Doctors Mayo,* my life had been indirectly linked with the clinic. Back when he was my professor and chief, Barcroft was also a trustee of the Wellcome Trust, the largest medical research charity in Great Britain, whose roots, remarkably enough, first grew in Minnesota with the encouragement of none other than William Worrall Mayo.

The story begins in 1853 with the birth of Henry Wellcome, cofounder of the international pharmaceutical company Burroughs, Wellcome, and Company (now GlaxoSmithKline). Wellcome grew up in Garden City near Rochester, Minnesota, where he learned the rudiments of pharmacy from an English chemist working in his uncle's drugstore. In 1870 Wellcome landed a job with a firm of pharmaceutical chemists in Rochester through his uncle's friend, W. W. Mayo, who urged the young man to go to college. After Wellcome graduated from the Philadelphia College of Pharmacy, he formed a new pharmaceutical firm in London with fellow American Silas Burroughs. They made their mark by manufacturing and marketing a compressed form of medicine pills that could be mass-produced for wide distribution. Knighted by King George V in 1932, Wellcome often returned to the United States and to Rochester. He always spoke with gratitude about W. W. Mayo, referring affectionately to the doctor and his famed sons as "my barefoot friends on the prairie" and saying he owed everything to the elder Mayo's inspiration, kindness, and advice. Henry Wellcome died the following year. Upon his death the Wellcome Trust was established.

My other early link to the Mayo Clinic was through my acquaintance with Sir Henry Dale, the Wellcome Trust's long-time chair. With William Creasy, president of Burroughs Wellcome Company–USA, Dale envisioned an extension of the trust in the United States called the Burroughs Wellcome Fund. Since its inception in 1955, the fund has focused its modest financial resources in selected areas to advance scientific knowledge. Mayo doesn't apply for funds, believing that this would be inappropriate, but other institutions in and around Rochester have. Since 1987, for instance, the Lake Crystal Wellcome Memorial Area Schools of the Minnesota Valley have served the communities of Lake Crystal, Vernon Center, Rapidan, Judson, and Garden City. In 1959, I crossed paths with Dale, who was visiting his former pupil, Charles Code, then chair of Mayo's physiology section. Unable to join Dale and Code, Barcroft asked me to accompany them to an appreciation ceremony in Garden City to relate the long association of Henry Wellcome and the Mayo Clinic.

Apart from the personal effect *The Doctors Mayo* had had on me, my excitement about my Mayo sabbatical derived from an affinity for the United States that I shared with many of my countrymen. Those of my generation knew the part that the immigrant Irish had played in the development of America. The very place where I was born, County Antrim in Northern Ireland, was also the ancestral home of Mark Twain, as well as six U.S. presidents: Andrew Jackson, Andrew Johnson, Chester A. Arthur, Grover Cleveland, William T. McKinley, and Theodore Roosevelt. Five other U.S. presidents also traced their roots to Ulster: James Polk, James Buchanan, Ulysses S. Grant, Benjamin Harrison, and Thomas Woodrow Wilson.

The famine caused by the Irish potato crop failures between 1845 and 1848 resulted in more than two million people (mostly Roman Catholic) leaving Ireland, the majority for the United States. But few people today realize that the Great Famine does not mark the beginning of the Irish in America. During the eighteenth century, three thousand to five thousand Ulster (Northern Ireland) Protestants, mostly men and Presbyterians, left Ireland for America each year, settling in New Hampshire and Maine. Ministers among the immigrants built up the Presbyterian Church in North America.

Although more than a quarter of Ireland's population in the eighteenth century was Protestant, the Anglo-Irish Anglicans made up only a minority. The majority of them were the Presbyterian settlers in Ulster and their descendants. The Scots-Irish, as they became known in the United States, left Ulster hoping for a better life in America. For one thing, they could avoid the penal laws of the Church of England. The laws not only decreed that members of all other religions in England, Ireland, Scotland, and Wales had to pay tithes to the Church of England, but they also prohibited burying the dead without the funeral service of the established church.

As many as 250,000 Scots-Irish Presbyterians left for America before the outbreak of the American Revolution, and they were among the first to call publicly and fight for independence from Great Britain. Indeed, the Declaration of Independence was written by the hand of an Ulsterman (Charles Thompson, secretary of the Continental Congress), printed by an Ulsterman (John Dunlop, founder of America's first successful daily newspaper, *The Pennsylvania Packet*), and first read in public by the son of an Ulsterman (Colonel John Nixon). The only signature on the Declaration for a month was that of John Hancock, president of the Second Continental Congress, whose ancestors were Presbyterians from Northern Ireland. By 1790, one-sixth of the three million citizens of the United States were of Irish birth or descent.

So many of my countrymen had made the crossing to America before me that I felt comfortable and excited about going to the United States—and, more specifically, about going to the Mayo Clinic to learn more about the cardiovascular system.

early Mayo experiences

With my sabbatical appointment secured at Mayo (and with a Fulbright traveling scholarship to pay my fare), Helen and I sailed for North America in September 1953 aboard the *Empress of France.* With us were our five-year-old daughter, Gillian Mary (born March 12, 1948), and our seventeen-month-old son, Roger Frederick John (born April 15, 1952). First I presented a paper on my research at an International Congress of Physiology in Montreal, which my new chief in the Mayo Clinic's physiology section, Earl Wood, also attended. This was my family's first visit to Montreal, and it occurred during the city's worst recorded heat wave. As we sweltered without air-conditioning in our hotel room, a gasoline truck crashed on the street outside, filling the hot air with the pungent odor of spilled gas and causing our son to develop laryngitis. We gladly evacuated the hotel for alternative accommodations in student quarters at the University of Montreal.

After the conference my family and I flew to Chicago and on to Rochester. I had no trouble obtaining a visa. In those days, priorities were based on the country of origin of the early immigrants to the United States, and since the Irish were such a large contingent, the only question when I applied to the U.S. consulate in Belfast was, "When do you wish to go?"

My first impression of Mayo centered on the friendliness of the staff, including senior members. A demonstration of this classic welcoming spirit happened just after our arrival, when eminent cardiologist Howard Burchell invited us to his home, where he and his wife entertained us, partly with their squawking parrot. Later, while the Burchells went on a three-week vacation, they insisted we move into their home. Young Roger received a postcard from Dr. Burchell during our stay: "Hope your parents are not restricting your activities and everyone is using everything at 301 8th Avenue and having fun. If you happen to twist the bird's neck, it would be OK by me. Regards to all." The Shepherd-Burchell friendship has continued for many years.

As I had anticipated, Earl Wood and Jeremy Swan, my former colleague then working with Wood, had assembled a stimulating group of trainees from both the United States and abroad to join them in their physiology laboratory. Many of our group wrote original papers during this exciting period. Our custom in the lab was to volunteer for one another's projects as control subjects for heart catheterization. No institutional review committee existed back then to approve the procedures, and no one refused to volunteer when his turn came. We were rewarded for volunteering by being paid for the amount of blood we lost during the procedures!

I recall having needles inserted into all available arteries in my limbs and a catheter in my heart. Each of us received multiple injections of the dye known as Evans blue, which we soon discovered took weeks to disappear from the blood. As a result, we all developed an ashen look that persisted. Later, working with scientists from the Eastman Kodak Research Laboratories, Earl Wood and I. J. Fox developed a new dye, indocyanine green. "Cardiogreen," as we called it, is rapidly excreted by the liver, so even repeated injections don't result in that cadaveric gray. To this day, this dye helps physicians throughout the world determine the amount of blood pumped out by the heart. It is also used to estimate blood flow in the liver.

Coincidentally, my year's appointment at the Mayo Clinic occurred during the heyday of McCarthyism, a period of intense anti-Communism in the United States named after its leading proponent, Republication senator Joseph McCarthy of Wisconsin. In 1950, having just been voted the worst member of the U.S. Senate by a poll of Washington correspondents, McCarthy began to warn that Communists had infiltrated virtually every institution in America. He claimed to have the names of the number-one Soviet espionage agent and many other Communists, from U.S. government officials to military officers to distinguished citizens in all walks of life. His most spectacular accusation was that George C. Marshall, former army chief of staff and secretary of state, was a traitor. General Marshall was exonerated, but the lesson was plain for all: If so eminent a person as Marshall could be attacked, no one was safe in the harsh light of the anti-Communist witch hunt. Indeed, I perceived among my laboratory colleagues a concern they might say something that, if repeated by others, could lead to false accusations. Though McCarthy never exposed a single Communist in the government or ever produced evidence to prove his accusations, he ruined many a career. We who lived through this period learned how tyrants can emerge in any society, scare honest citizens, and inhibit democratic principles.

Toward the end of my sabbatical year at Mayo, I was invited to spend a second year. The offer was attractive, but Queen's University needed me to resume my teaching and research in Belfast. And so in September 1954 we booked our return passage from New York on the *Queen Mary*. Our journey back to Ireland was memorable, for ocean liners of this time, including the well-known *Queen Mary,* had no stabilizers to help minimize the roll caused by the Atlantic's Gulf stream. The ship rolled slowly almost forty-five degrees to starboard, and just as you began to wonder whether it would recover, it shook violently and moved slowly forty-five degrees to port. All of the Shepherd family became severely seasick, and we were glad indeed to reach port. Many years later, when I took my family back for a visit on the *Queen Mary,* which had been dry-docked as a tourist attraction in Long Beach, California, since her retirement in 1967, we all recalled our misery on that earlier voyage.

In 1955, a year after my return to Queen's University, I received a formal invitation to join the Mayo Clinic staff in the physiology section. What to do? I was by now a tenured faculty member at Queen's with the title of reader, a position next in line to the head of the department, the only person named professor. I had also been appointed consultant physiologist to the Northern Ireland Hospitals Authority, though without additional stipend.

Helen and I decided to approach the matter logically. We devised a system to compare the advantages of Mayo with those of Queen's. We thought of all the categories we could: stipend, housing, schooling for children, and more. We then rated each choice in all the categories, added up the points, made our decision, and went to bed—and the next morning changed the grading system! Finally, we decided with regret to decline the Mayo offer. We made our decision primarily because we enjoyed being close to our families, because our children had access to excellent schools close at hand, and because I enjoyed my research at Queen's University with a stimulating group of colleagues.

Shortly after Helen and I decided to remain in Ireland, I was awarded an Anglo-French Medical Exchange Bursary by the National Institute of

Hygiene of France to study for a few months at the Boûcicaut Hospital in Paris. I selected this site because it too was involved in heart catheterization. In this time, I learned more about French customs than medicine. When, for instance, I did not get my turn with my French associates to conduct cardiac procedures on the patients, I learned that each of them had earned that privilege by bringing flowers to my chief's secretary, rumored to be his mistress. After they advised me to do as they did, I too delivered flowers to the woman and achieved my proper turn in the rotations.

back to Mayo

I returned from Paris to my department at Queen's University in 1956, the year I was awarded the doctor of science degree. My two years of successful research on the heart and circulation after returning to Queen's from Mayo, plus a decade's worth of other research, had earned me the degree, for which there is no written or oral examination. The department chair first decides whether a candidate's published papers merit the degree. If so, he suggests a formal application to the appropriate university authorities. This approved, the department chair proposes two external examiners to review the papers and make their recommendation to the university, which is final. (In my earlier years, the word was that publications were weighed when you were considered for academic promotion. When we requested reprints of our published papers, we had the option to order them with or without covers. We always ordered them with covers!)

Soon after my return from Paris, I received a second invitation to join the staff of the Mayo Clinic. Would I reconsider my decision of the year before? This time, for no different reasons than before, Helen and I chose to accept—and we never regretted the decision.

Of course, Jeremy Swan's presence in the physiology section at Mayo was an important factor in my decision to return to Rochester in 1957. Swan was born in Sligo, near the cliff-rimmed Ben Bulben Mountain, a mecca for fans of W. B. Yeats. (As one of those fans, I occasionally visit the little churchyard at Drumcliffe where the poet is buried. His grave bears a simple limestone slab inscribed, "Cast a cold eye on Life and Death, Horseman pass by.") Swan's parents were physicians, and soon after Jeremy completed his medical degree at the University of London, he was appointed a research fellow in physiology at the University of London. He worked for a doctorate at St. Thomas Hospital under my mentor, Henry Barcroft, then with the chair of St. Thomas's physiology department. Swan continued Barcroft's studies of the sympathetic nerves to the blood vessels of the limbs in humans by looking at the action of norepinephrine and epinephrine on the circulation to skeletal muscles and skin. (The Swedish physiologist Ulf von Euler, who shared the Nobel Prize in physiology or medicine in 1970, had demonstrated in 1946 that norepinephrine was the mediator of excitatory sympathetic impulses.) Swan also made original studies on patients with tumors of the suprarenal glands, known as pheochromocytomas, which cause high arterial blood pressure by secreting these substances into the circulation. After completing his doctorate in 1951, Swan became a research associate and later a staff member in the Mayo Clinic's physiology section.

During his years in Rochester, Swan played a key role in establishing the Rochester Civic Theatre and even acted in some of the plays. (Acting was never my forte. My only experience consisted of playing the female Thisby in a high school production of Shakespeare's *A Midsummer Night's Dream,* reciting such lines as, "O wall, full often has thou heard my moans, / For parting my fair Pyramus and me." To which Pyramus responded, "Oh, kiss me through the hole of this vile wall," and I replied, "I kiss the wall's hole, not your lips at all." Shakespeare notwithstanding, you can imagine the ribbing I took!)

At the end of my final lecture to the medical students at Queen's University, shortly before my family and I returned to the United States, I received a silver goblet with the inscription "From All the Queen's 'Meds'—1957."

life in a new land

In September 1957, my family and I embarked on the *S.S. America* for the voyage from Ireland to a new life in America. Our return journey to Rochester, Minnesota, and the Mayo Clinic began by train from Belfast to southern Ireland and continued by ship from the port of Cobh (the same port from which the *Titanic* left on her fateful maiden voyage in 1912) to the port of New York. Helen, Gillian, Roger, and I boarded the *America,* and in the rough September seas of the Atlantic Ocean her bow and stern moved thirty to forty feet up and down for much of the five-day voyage. As we walked her decks, we clung to the hand ropes strung everywhere. Eating was next to impossible. The edges of the dining room tables had hinged turn-ups, which prevented plates, cutlery, and stemware from ending on our laps. After we arrived in New York City, our son, Roger, then five years old, walked just as he had onboard—weaving from side to side.

We decided to spend a few days in New York before proceeding to Rochester. One day, when I took my family to the Waldorf-Astoria Hotel for lunch, our daughter, Gillian, then eight, cautioned her brother, "You don't do a thing for yourself in this hotel." While we were having lunch, Roger had to go to the restroom. "The attendant in there was upset with me because I did not flush the toilet," he told us after he emerged. "But I was just behaving the way my sister told me I should!"

Upon reaching Rochester, we moved into a house that Jeremy Swan had rented for us, which gave us time in which to look for a permanent home. Helen and I soon found a new house that we liked in an attractive area of Rochester, about a block from the Mayo Foundation House. With a loan from the clinic, we bought the house and moved in. At that time, the clinic provided home loans for staff members payable over time at below-market interest. The terms were so favorable that we were later able to delay payments while our children attended prep school and college. (Since Helen and I had gone to private preparatory schools in Ireland, we decided our children would do the same. Thus, Gillian attended the Baldwin Schools for Girls in Pennsylvania and Roger attended Choate School in Connecticut. Of the three preparatory schools for girls in the mainline area of Philadelphia—Baldwin, Irwin, and Shipley—the buzz was Baldwin for brains, Irwin for games, and Shipley for dames!)

Helen and I soon began to play host to family visiting from Ireland, including my parents and Aunt Lena. My father, who had always displayed his Princeton Theological Seminary shield in a prominent place in his home, particularly enjoyed his return to the United States. (He later presented the shield to me.) Back then, and perhaps still today, visitors to America had to sign a form stating that they would not engage in illegal activities before obtaining a visa. I received an urgent message from my mother before her visit; she understood that she should not engage in prostitution, but she wondered what might be involved in "moral turpitude"!

Helen's widowed mother also came to visit; with her only child and grandchildren so far away, she was lonely. We subsequently vowed to return with our children to Ireland every August. We would visit Helen's mother and other of her relatives, as well as the large contingent of Shepherds who assembled each August on the Atlantic coast in County Donegal.

But first I set about obtaining my medical license in Minnesota. Without it I could not conduct research on patients. The examination was in two parts, first a written test on basic medical sciences, then an oral exam. At the latter the examiner said to me, "So *you* are the physiologist." Because I was principally a researcher and wouldn't be diagnosing or treating patients, he made the rest of the exam easy. To maintain my license, I was required to become a U.S. citizen within five years, which I did.

an unexpected career decision

With Minnesota medical license in hand, I was ready to begin my own research program at Mayo, and I set about recruiting talented young research fellows to work with me. Within months of my arrival at the clinic, however, I was faced with another major career choice. The University of Toronto was offering me a tenured professorship in its medical research department, funded by the Canadian Heart Association. Suddenly I had to decide whether to leave the remarkable institution I had just joined.

The proposal was made by American physiologist Charles Herbert Best, famed for his discovery of insulin in 1921 with Frederick Grant Banting while working in the University of Toronto laboratories of John Macleod. Banting and Macleod had received the Nobel Prize in physiology or medicine in 1923. Recognizing that Best should have been his cowinner, Banting voluntarily shared his portion of the cash award with Best. The university created the Banting and Best Department of Medical Research that same year. Best, who succeeded Banting as the department's director, discovered the vitamin choline and the enzyme histaminase, and was the first to introduce anticoagulants in the treatment of thrombosis.

Helen and I had first met Charles Best in July 1957, when he and his wife visited Northern Ireland to explore her Irish heritage. Upon settling in his hotel room, Best studied the phone book and found it full of listings for Mahon, his wife's maiden name. In his systematic way, he began to telephone each one in turn. His third call connected him with a Roman Catholic priest, who demanded to know why he was calling. "I will have you know, my good man, that I am a member of the Papal Academy of Sciences," Best replied. The priest naturally assumed that, despite Best's Canadian accent, the caller was a Protestant Orangeman playing a joke on him—for the date was July 12. (For Best, July 12 held little significance, but in Ireland the date commemorates the defeat of the Catholic King James II of England in 1690 by the mostly mercenary forces of his son-in-law, the Protestant William of Orange, at the Battle of the Boyne River in Ireland. Each year since on July 12, the Orangemen have marched in Northern Ireland to drums and bagpipes to celebrate the victory over Catholicism. The irony, of course, is that a Protestant, armed with the blessing of the pope, went into battle against a Catholic!)

After Best told his story a day or so later in the physiology department at

Queen's University, a few of us made inquiries into his wife's family connections. We learned they were likely in Londonderry. A colleague and I offered to drive the Bests to Derry, on the river Foyle in the northwest part of Northern Ireland, accompanied by our wives. Beforehand, I phoned the mayor of Derry to tell him that an eminent man of medicine would be visiting his city. He agreed to host a luncheon in Derry's historic Guildhall. We arrived to find that the mayor also had invited some twenty other guests, though none was a physician or scientist. Just before he rose to welcome the Bests, the mayor turned to me and whispered, "Where does he come from, what does he do, and why is he famous?" I whispered back, "An outstanding physiologist from Toronto who discovered insulin and should have been a cowinner of the Nobel Prize." To my dismay, the mayor whispered back, "What is insulin and what does it do?" I did my best to explain insulin in the next few seconds, but he failed to grasp its significance. During the introduction, the mayor looked at me and asked, "Professor Best is a physiol-*what*?"

Charles Best offered me the tenured professorship in 1958 at the University of Toronto at the same time he invited me to deliver a lecture, all expenses paid. Helen and I enjoyed our reunion with the Bests and the time we spent with members of my deceased Uncle Harry's family. I was also duly impressed with Best's excellent laboratory facilities. But I declined his generous offer. Even though tenure was not offered at Mayo Clinic, I had been assured upon my arrival there that if my performance were satisfactory I could expect to stay until I turned sixty-five, the compulsory age of retirement. I simply did not wish to miss the opportunities and challenges in the constructive, stimulating, and friendly atmosphere of the Mayo Clinic.

(I received a similar offer in 1963, some six years after I came to Mayo, when my alma mater, Queen's University, approached me to become chair of its physiology department. I discussed my dilemma with my colleague and close friend, Ward Fowler, who took the matter to the clinic's leaders. I am still grateful for the way they handled this. The senior administrator, Slade Schuster, told me he knew about the offer and understood my dilemma. Perhaps, he suggested, my decision would be made easier if I knew what Mayo had in mind for me in the future: I would be invited to become director for research and to join Mayo's board of governors and its board of trustees.)

Thus my decision to stay at the Mayo Clinic was made. What would become a forty-five-year career in clinical research at the renowned institution had at last begun in earnest.

2 directing Mayo research

When I joined the staff of the Mayo Clinic in 1957, it marked the beginning of a long and satisfying career for me in medical research in the section of physiology. Over the course of four decades, I worked with talented Mayo research fellows – forty in all – studying the human cardiovascular system. My research efforts have resulted in the publication of more than eight books as well as 236 scientific papers and scores of abstracts. In addition to editing the journal News in Physiological Sciences, *I served on the editorial boards of sixteen research journals.*

In 1962 I became a full professor of physiology and, four years later, chair of the clinic's department of physiology and biophysics. The 1960s and 1970s encompassed an extraordinary period of change for Mayo, and, as its first director for research during that time, I worked with my colleagues throughout the clinic to improve Mayo's research resources, both physical and financial. Our accomplishments included defining criteria for extramural research funding from such organizations as the National Institutes of Health; establishing a much-needed pharmacology department; and creating state-of-the-art Mayo research facilities, particularly the Guggenheim and Hilton Buildings at Mayo Rochester. Our work during those years subsequently served as the foundation for research programs at Mayo's newly established Jacksonville and Scottsdale clinics as well.

My own research goals at Mayo and my contributions as director for research were achieved in a much greater context, of course – the context of the clinic's long-standing history of research, beginning modestly after the turn of the twentieth century in a barn behind the house of Mayo's pioneering pathologist, Louis B. Wilson.

Mayo's early research

Louis B. Wilson, who joined the Mayo Clinic in 1905, became internationally known for developing the frozen-section diagnostic technique. This biopsy procedure allows pathologists to examine tiny tissue samples while patients are undergoing surgery and then to report the diagnostic results instantly to the surgeon. Wilson devised the technique in response to William James Mayo's desire to see whether and to what extent his patients had cancer while they were still on the operating table.

Shortly after joining the clinic, Wilson asked Dr. Will what his budget for research would be. Dr. Will replied that when Wilson wanted something, he should simply ask and he would get it. How the world has changed! Wilson's first research building was a barn built in 1908 behind his house for $500. It housed two operating rooms and four rooms for animals. In six years the laboratory moved to the first building designed for the Mayos' group practice of medicine. Completed in 1914, with the words "Mayo Clinic" inscribed over the main doors, the building was finished with red Pennsylvania brick and trimmed with Missouri marble. The red-brick building was adjacent to the Kahler Hotel, but when hotel guests complained about barking dogs housed at the lab, the facility moved three miles southwest of Rochester to forty acres of land donated by Charles Mayo. The new building seemed far from the rest of the clinic, but Wilson's colleague Frank C. Mann defended the location, saying it prevented investigators from becoming the "handmaidens" of the clinicians. When the building burned to the ground, it was rebuilt for $80,000 on the same site and opened in 1924 as the Institute for Experimental Medicine with a staff of nine researchers and twenty technicians. Its budget was $100,000 a year.

Leonard Roundtree oversaw clinical research at Mayo during the 1920s. With Russell Wilder, he formed a clinical research unit at Saint Marys Hospital, which did excellent work on diabetes, insulin therapy, and hyperparathyroidism. However, the hospital research unit became a clinic independent of Mayo as a whole, contrary to the clinic's philosophy of collaboration. When in 1930 the unit sought to develop a laboratory for animal experimentation to complement human studies, Mayo's board of governors voted to dissolve it.

From this episode the Mayo Clinic learned that research can neither stand alone nor be confined to a few who become isolated from their peers. On the principle that research must be integrated with education and medical practice, Mayo abandoned the Institute for Experimental Medicine after World War II and replaced it with the Medical Sciences Building, closer to the clinical buildings in downtown Rochester.

Throughout the 1930s and the 1940s, Mayo participated in rapid advancements in aviation medicine. Airplane designers had the know-how to build planes that could fly higher above the earth, but needed to know how pilots could be prevented from blacking out from a lack of oxygen when they reached the thin atmosphere of high altitudes. Among those seeking a solution was William Randolph Lovelace II, who became a Mayo fellow and surgical resident in 1935. In collaboration with Walter Boothby and Arthur Bulbulian, then director of the Mayo Medical Museum, Lovelace designed a device in 1938 known as the BLB (for Boothby, Lovelace, and Bulbulian) inhalation apparatus. Placed on the aviator's nose, the apparatus delivered oxygen from a portable tank. Of great value to aviators, including fighter pilots, the device also benefited earthbound patients requiring oxygen therapy.

The potential military value of the BLB mask was immediately apparent. Quietly produced in great quantities, many of the masks were shipped to England in 1939 after war broke out between Germany and Great Britain. RAF fighter pilots relied on the advantage the BLB masks gave them during the Battle of Britain in 1940, when they foiled German plans to invade England. President Franklin D. Roosevelt awarded the National Aeronautics Association's Collier Trophy to Boothby, Lovelace, and Harry Armstrong, chief of the aeromedical laboratory at Wright-Patterson Field in Dayton, Ohio, for their work in developing the BLB mask.

Lovelace was named to head Mayo's general surgery section in 1941, but with war imminent he joined the army air corps and succeeded Armstrong as chief of the aeromedical lab at Wright-Patterson Field. Lovelace intended to prove the effectiveness of the BLB mask to the air force, which he did by jumping with the mask from 40,200 feet. In the process he set a world's record for a parachute jump—and suffered long-lasting effects of frostbite when his parachute ripped the glove from his hand. The demonstration led to the saving of countless aviators' lives during WWII. Lovelace returned to Mayo as a surgical consultant but left again in 1947 to establish the Lovelace Foundation in Albuquerque, New Mexico. Later, he headed the physical selection team that picked NASA's first Project Mercury astronauts and assumed prime responsibility for keeping the astronauts functioning effectively during their space flights.

Although the British had been fighting the Axis powers for more than two years, the war for the United States began December 7, 1941, when the Japanese launched their surprise attack on the U.S. Pacific fleet at Pearl Harbor. Within months, Mayo had formed an aeromedical unit—organized by Charles Code, E. J. Baldes, and Walter Boothby—and offered its services to the military for one dollar a year. The aeromedical unit's purpose was to design and build a human centrifuge that would simulate the blackouts aviators experienced in high-powered airplanes during high-speed turns and when pulling out of dives. Baldes, head of the Mayo biophysics section, obtained two forty-ton flywheels from a brewery out East to power parts salvaged from a junked Chrysler. The establishment of the aeromedical unit in 1942 coincided with the construction of Mayo's centrifuge, the first of its type. When I first came to Mayo on sabbatical from Queen's University in 1953, someone told me that Wood recommended a ride on the human centrifuge before breakfast as a good way to wake up. I concluded from my own experience that I greatly preferred coffee!

My future chief in Mayo's physiology section, Earl Wood, was persuaded to leave his research at Harvard University in 1942 and return home to Minnesota to study what caused pilots to black out. He learned they did so because the mechanical forces of high-speed dives and sharp turns deprived their brains of blood. Among Wood's colleagues working to develop antiblackout technology was famed Minnesota aviator Charles A. Lindbergh. After three years of work—aided by the expertise of David Clark from Worcester, Massachusetts, who manufactured brassieres and corsets—the Mayo team designed a G-suit that combated blackouts during high-speed dives. Clark's firm later made the space suit worn by the astronauts.

studying the human cardiovascular system

Mayo had long been a center of important cardiac studies thanks to Jesse Edwards, who had established a world-class cardiac pathology department at the clinic. (With his Mayo colleague Robert Fontana, Edwards later wrote the 1962 classic *Congenital Heart Disease: A Review of 357 Cases Studied Pathologically.*) During and after WWII, Earl Wood's studies on Mayo's human centrifuge involved developing methods to continuously measure arterial blood pressure and the oxygen content of the blood, as well as creating techniques to prevent the loss of consciousness during high gravitational forces. Wood applied this experience to the evaluation of patients with cardiac diseases by comparing their test results with those of normal volunteer subjects, including me.

The Mayo Clinic originally conducted aviation research in a three-story building built in 1941 in downtown Rochester for the Institute for Experimental Medicine. Responding to the need for larger research facilities after World War II, Mayo began construction in 1949 of an addition immediately south of the original structure that more than doubled the size of the facility. Vannevar Bush of the Carnegie Institute spoke in 1952 at the dedication of the renamed Medical Sciences Building, which the Minnesota Society of Architects cited for its design excellence. (Mayo later added laboratories for anatomy, biochemistry, biophysics, pathology, physiology, and surgical work.) The Medical Sciences Building also included an engineering section that custom-built laboratory equipment for Mayo scientists, as well as an assembly hall for lectures and demonstrations named for Frank C. Mann, Mayo's research pioneer.

Since it was only a short walk from the clinical practice buildings, the Medical Sciences Building gave clinicians and scientists even more opportunities for collaboration than before. As the cardiac surgeons developed more methods for treating patients with congenital or acquired heart diseases, for instance, Mayo's cardiologists sent more patients to the Medical Sciences Building for diagnostic heart catheterization. The patients began to include children with congenital heart disease. Under Earl Wood's leadership, specialists in the physiology department excelled in studying systemic and pulmonary circulation, making many advances in the diagnosis and management of many forms of heart disease. In the mid-1950s, for example, Wood and Jeremy Swan learned to diagnose congenital and acquired forms of heart disease by injecting a dye into the heart and measuring blood pressure and flow. After I joined them in the heart-catheterization laboratory, we conducted and published the results of many other investigations.

On one occasion soon after I joined Mayo, I conducted the catheterization procedure in a woman with severe heart failure in a room in the Medical Sciences Building. When her heart stopped beating, we summoned a surgeon, who attempted to restart it. Even though the cardiac surgeon arrived quickly to open her chest and massage her heart, she died. This experience—together with the need for a staff anesthesiologist to assist with procedures in children—emphasized that the time had come to move these complex procedures to Saint Marys Hospital, where cardiac surgery, cardiac anesthesia, and pediatric cardiology services were located in-house.

Swan became head of the new cardiac-catheterization laboratory at Saint Marys Hospital in 1960. He had just returned from two months at the Karolinska Institute in Stockholm, where he had become skilled in angiocardiography. The technique involves using an x-ray contrast dye to diagnose congenital heart malformations. But in 1965, after concluding he could contribute more as a cardiologist than as a physiologist, Swan moved to Cedar Sinai Hospital in Los Angeles, where he developed an outstanding clinical practice. Based on his experiences in heart catheterization at Mayo, Swan developed with his colleague Willy Ganz a flow-directed, balloon-tipped catheter that could "float" into the human pulmonary artery. Introduced in 1970, the new device made catheterization of the right side of the heart a practical and safe procedure at bedside, in the anesthesia suite, operating room, or intensive care unit, as well as in the catheterization laboratory.

heart surgery at Mayo

Open-heart surgery came of age at the Mayo Clinic in the mid-1950s. Working with heart surgeon John Kirklin and engineer Richard Jones, David Donald was a key contributor to the development of a heart-lung machine, which permitted surgeons to operate on nonbeating hearts. The device was integral not only to surgeries to correct congenital and acquired heart diseases, but also to the cardiac bypass procedure that Kirklin was then perfecting. Trained in Scotland as a veterinarian, Donald used his surgical skills to create common human cardiac defects in dogs. Kirklin then performed a bypass, stopped the animals' defective hearts from beating, and with Donald's help made the necessary repairs.

Only when satisfied that the bypass worked well in dogs did Kirklin proceed to perform the procedure on humans. With Donald assisting him, Kirklin performed the first open-heart surgery at Mayo on March 22, 1955. Rochester Methodist Hospital was one of the first in the world to use the Mayo-Gibbon mechanical pump-oxygenator for a successful operation inside the heart. This remarkable device was demonstrated at Methodist Hospital on September 12, 1955, before a television audience estimated at six to nine million, the first nationally televised broadcast to originate from Rochester. Mayo afterward released the rights for the Mayo-Gibbon mechanical pump-oxygenator to a commercial manufacturer for international distribution. After additional experience with human patients showed everything proceeding satisfactorily, Mayo offered Donald a staff appointment in surgical research.

The remarkable collaboration between heart surgeon John Kirklin and veterinarian David Donald might not have occurred without an event in which I played a part. I had met Donald during my first stint at Mayo in 1953, the year I began my sabbatical from Queen's University. Recently married to a medical technician at Mayo, Donald and his bride had decided to return to Scotland and in fact had purchased their airline tickets. Before making the journey, however, they went camping in Florida's Okefenokee Swamp. Both loved rugged outdoor challenges. Eager to get the heart-surgery program under way, Kirklin wanted Donald to cancel his plans and return to Rochester to assist him. Since Donald and I had become close friends,

Kirklin asked me to find Donald and persuade him to return. This was no easy task. Just try to find someone camping amid alligators in a swamp! But I made the trip to Florida and, with help from the local police, found the Donalds. Fortunately for Mayo, Donald agreed to return.

David Donald first came to Mayo after learning that members of the surgical research section were studying cardiac arrhythmia in dogs. Back in Scotland, Donald had demonstrated at the racetracks that horses were liable during races to develop arrhythmia. He and I quickly became friends, in part perhaps because we shared a common culture and upbringing. Each of us was familiar with the popularity of greyhound racing in Ireland and Scotland, and we appreciated the speed and energy required of the dogs. How, we wondered, would they perform in the absence of the nervous control of their hearts?

Donald and I approached a veterinary consultant at the nearest greyhound racetrack, in Elk Point, South Dakota, and he agreed to join our inquiry. Unlike thoroughbred horses, greyhounds diminish in value once they cease to win, so we were able to buy a few over-the-hill racers for $25 each. To answer our question, we timed them on the race circuit, then we brought them to Rochester, where Donald performed surgical denervation of their hearts. After they recovered, we brought the dogs back to Elk Point and raced them again, comparing their times with those recorded before surgery. The two racing times were surprisingly close.

The denervated heart performs so well because it becomes increasingly sensitive to circulating substances, which augment its rate and force of contraction. When the action of these substances was blocked in the greyhounds after their hearts were denervated, their racing times were much diminished. Our findings indicated that transplanted hearts in humans, if not immunologically rejected, would perform satisfactorily and meet everyday stresses, including muscular exercise. In fact, our conclusions were subsequently confirmed. The first human heart transplant at Mayo occurred in 1988.

working with research fellows

After Mayo moved the heart catheterization unit to Saint Marys Hospital, I was free to engage full-time in research at the Medical Sciences Building. One of the most rewarding consequences of my almost fifty years of studying the cardiovascular system was the opportunity to work with research fellows and to enjoy following their subsequent careers.

The designation "Mayo fellow" has a venerable history. Will Mayo wished to indicate that those in training in the Mayo Graduate School were neither "yes-men" nor flunkies for the permanent staff. Mayo researcher and pathologist Louis B. Wilson (who in 1905 had developed the frozen-section biopsy technique) suggested the term *fellow* from the Anglo-Saxon *felawe,* meaning comrade or companion. Thus "fellow of the Mayo Clinic" was coined.

Many of the young men and women from overseas who train at Mayo for an academic career in their own countries come for a second benefit: to attain what has been nicknamed the B.T.A. ("Been to America") degree! In addition to fellows from the United States, I have worked with those from Australia, Belgium, Canada, China, Denmark, England, France, Germany, Greece, Holland, Ireland, Israel, Italy, the Soviet Union, Sweden, and Yugoslavia—a total of forty fellows. During one period I simultaneously mentored a sophisticated Italian who spoke no English, a proper Oxford-educated Englishman, and an Australian with a decidedly down-under accent. All three occupied a single office. The English that Ettore Ambrosioni, my Italian colleague, learned from the other two fellows, Webb Peploe and David Brender, as well as from my own soft Irish tongue, had a unique international flavor, to say the least.

I worked with my first and second fellows, Herbert Semler and Robert Marshall, in the late 1950s. I had published studies in 1953 with colleagues in Belfast showing that the substance acetylcholine, which is released from certain nerves in the body, causes the vessels controlling blood flow to the hand and forearm to dilate. When I joined Mayo in 1957, I decided to test the effect of acetylcholine on the blood vessels in human lungs. (In 1953 Marshall and I, together with another colleague in the physiology department at Queen's, had studied a rare blood factor in patients who, when exposed to severe cold, experienced the clotting of blood in their fingers, which, of course, stopped the flow. The condition quickly reversed when they warmed their fingers.) Marshall had just completed a fellowship in Australia, and together with Earl Wood, Fred Helmholz, and Herbert Semler, we published a series of papers in 1959 on our studies of patients with constricted blood vessels controlling flow to the lungs. The constricted flow caused the right side of the heart to fail from the increased stress of pumping blood returned through the constricted vessels. We demonstrated that infusing acetylcholine into the main pulmonary artery caused the constricted vessels to relax—and the patients to feel much better.

The results of these studies perplexed us, however, since earlier studies of isolated blood vessels had demonstrated that exposure to acetylcholine caused them to contract. The mystery was not explained until many years later. During the late 1950s, the usual practice was to cut spiral strips from the blood vessels, which consequently damaged the endothelium, the layer of cells lining the insides of the vessels. In 1980, Robert F. Furchgott and J. V. Zawadzki used circular strips but kept the lining of the endothelium intact. They found that acetylcholine acted on the endothelial cells to cause the release of what they termed endothelium-derived relaxing factor, or EDRF. The release of EDRF—later shown to be nitric oxide—resulted in the relaxation of the smooth muscle of the intact circular strips. With Louis Ignarro of the University of California in Los Angeles and Ferid Murad of the University of Texas in Houston, Furchgott received the Nobel Prize for physiology or medicine in 1998 for the discovery that nitric oxide signals the cardiovascular system to relax blood vessels.

Today, patients with constricted blood vessels in the lungs get relief from inhaling nitric oxide. Nitric oxide also affects the endothelial cells of blood vessels elsewhere in the human body. This is the basis of the impotence treatment Viagra, which enhances the formation of nitric oxide in the vessels of the penis, thus increasing the blood flow in response to sexual stimulation.

(Paul Vanhoutte, a former fellow and colleague, showed that the endothelium forms another substance that causes the vessels to dilate. He called it endothelium-derived hyperpolarizing factor—EDHF—but its identity is still unknown. Subsequent studies worldwide have shown that endothelium can form both relaxing and contracting factors. The relaxing factors seem to predominate in health, while the contracting factors are preeminent in circulatory diseases. As an example, patients with high blood pressure fail to form nitric oxide in their arterial blood vessels.)

Herbert Semler, my first fellow, returned to medical practice in Portland, Oregon. In 1977 he and his wife, Shirley, provided funds to the Mayo Foundation to endow a scholarship in Mayo Medical School. My second fellow, Robert Marshall, and I had coauthored fourteen published papers on the cardiovascular system when he became professor of medicine and head of cardiology at West Virginia University's newly established medical school in Morgantown. Later, we joined forces to write the 1968 book *Cardiac Function in Health and Disease.*

My third fellow was Yang Wang, a graduate of Beijing University. Together with Marshall, we studied the effects on the heart and circulation of changes in posture and graded exercise in normal young humans and in dogs. Altogether, we published five papers between 1960 and 1962. Wang left Mayo to join the cardiology department at the University of Minnesota Medical School.

While I cannot profile each of my forty research fellows, several bear special mention. In the 1960s Norman Browse and Tore Strandell stand out.

Norman Leslie Browse, a graduate of Saint Bartholomew's Hospital Medical School and a lecturer in surgery at the Westminster Hospital in London, joined me as a research associate in 1964. With his surgical interest and skills in the venous system, Browse worked with me to study various reflex mechanisms governing this system. On the basis of his research at Mayo, Browse was selected by the Royal College of Surgeons to give the renowned Arris and Gale Lecture in November 1965. This was later published in the *Annals of the Royal College of Surgeons* as "The Veins and Cardiovascular Reflexes." He became professor of vascular surgery at St. Thomas's Hospital in 1972 and published his textbook, *Diseases of the Veins,* in 1988.

Browse changed the initials after his name from "FRCS" (fellow of the Royal College of Surgeons) to "PRCS" (president) after his election as leader of the Royal College. He was knighted in 1994, and I enjoyed visiting Sir Norman and Lady Jeanne Browse, also a physician, in the regal presidential apartment of the Royal College. In 1993 I nominated Browse for the Mayo Distinguished Alumnus Award, which he received at Mayo graduation ceremonies in May of that year. Two years later, in 1995, Sir Norman Leslie Browse became an honorary fellow in the American College of Surgeons. In the citation, John E. Connolly of Irvine, California, noted that Sir Norman was a "superb technical surgeon who obtains excellent results especially in the field of vascular surgery," adding that his mentors included the distinguished English surgeons James Paterson Ross, John Kinmonth, Harold Ellis, and Roy Calne, and, in America, "the distinguished physiologist John Shepherd."

Tore Strandell followed Browse to join me in 1965. Strandell was one in a series of fellows from Stockholm; he and Sture Bevegård, Anders Melcher, and Lars-Erik Lindblad were specialists in clinical physiology, most of whom trained with Torgny Sjöstrand, the founder of clinical physiology at Karolinska Hospital. All became department heads at hospitals in Stockholm.

Strandell earned his medical and doctorate degrees at the Karolinska Institute; the title of his thesis was *Central Circulation in Healthy Elderly Men.* He studied his subjects (the oldest were eighty-three) through right-heart catheterization at rest and during exercise. During his year at Mayo, we investigated the effect in humans of increased sympathetic activity on the blood flow to active forearm muscles. On his return to Stockholm, Strandell became head of the Department of Clinical Physiology at the Epidemiological

Hospital. Such departments originated in Sweden as diagnostic laboratories for the study of heart, lung, and blood vessel function. In addition to testing patients with different infections, Strandell developed with his surgical colleagues a technique to study the streamlining of portal-vein blood flow and to measure dual liver blood flow in awake patients. He achieved this by inserting multiple catheters into the umbilical vein.

In 1972, when his laboratory closed, Strandell moved to Sankt Eriks Hospital. This too closed in 1986, so he moved to Stockholm's Sabbatsbergs Hospital, which closed in 1993. Thus he claimed to be the most closed-down clinical physiologist in the world!

Strandell started a private laboratory in clinical physiology in Stockholm in 1981, but it had no facilities to monitor patients with disturbed sleep, which he was interested in researching and from which he himself suffered. Encouraged by a visit in 1983 to Mayo's Sleep Disorder Center, he started a section to study snoring and sleep apnea in his laboratory and at Sabbatsbergs Hospital. He developed multiple ambulatory tests to monitor patients with sleep apnea. He recruited retired heads of hospital laboratories in Sweden to assist him, including Sture Bevegård, who had joined me as a fellow at Mayo in 1963. (We had concentrated on factors regulating the circulation during physical exercise in man.) Strandell's 1991 book on snoring for patients and health care providers soon established him as an expert in sleep apnea. Today more sleep tests are performed at his laboratory than at all the hospitals in Stockholm.

It's interesting to note that Tore Strandell is a descendant of Carl Linnaeus, the famous eighteenth-century Swedish naturalist. Linnaeus, who had studied medicine and natural science, introduced binomial nomenclature, a system of information storage and retrieval, first for plants, then for animals. Strandell's father inherited Linnaeus's papers and sold the collection in 1967 to the Hunt Institute for Botanical Documentation at Carnegie-Mellon University in Pittsburgh, and most of it is now housed in the Strandell Room there.

During my years at Queen's University, my colleagues and I demonstrated the importance of receptors in the heart and lungs, in addition to those in the arteries to the brain and in the aorta, to the regulation of reflexes in the cardiovascular system. Five Mayo fellows helped continue these studies in animals in the 1970s: Anthony Edis from Australia (who later joined the surgical staff at Mayo, then returned to practice in Perth), Norbert Ott from Germany, Conrad Pelletier from Canada, Peter Thorén from Sweden, and Giuseppe Mancia from Italy. Mancia is now the acknowledged expert on the arterial baroreflexes and other cardiovascular reflexes governing the circulatory system in normal humans and those with mild and severe essential hypertension.

Two of my fellows during this time won the Young Investigators Award presented by the American College of Cardiology on the basis of their research at Mayo: Conrad Pelletier in 1972, and Paul Vanhoutte the next year, from the University of Ghent. Peter Thorén was the second-place winner in 1975.

As it happened, four of my Mayo fellows came from Flanders. In addition to Paul Vanhoutte they are Denis Clement, Daniel Duprez, and Raymond Verhaeghe. These men have furthered our knowledge of the reflex and local mechanisms that regulate circulation. Clement was dean of the medical school in Ghent, Belgium, and head of the Department of Cardiology and Angiology at University Hospital. Duprez was a member of the same department. Verhaeghe is a physician and professor at the Universitaire Ziekenhuizen in Leuven. Vanhoutte became director of research and development at the Institut De Recherches Internationales Servier in Nueilly-sur-Seine Cedex, France, and now resides in Hong Kong.

Paul Vanhoutte was at Mayo on three separate occasions, the first time as a research assistant in 1968 and 1969. A graduate of the State Medical School in Ghent, Vanhoutte developed his interest in blood vessels on the basis of the classic experiments conducted at his medical school by Corneel Heymans. (Heymans discovered the existence of chemoreflexes to control breathing, for which he received the Nobel Prize in physiology or medicine in 1938.) Vanhoutte's first research project at the University of Ghent was on the role of receptors in the main arteries of the neck and the aorta in dogs in regulating arterial blood pressure. His chief, the head of the Department of Normal and Pathological Physiology, Isodore Leusen, was a Mayo alumnus who knew of my similar studies and recommended Vanhoutte for Mayo.

Vanhoutte returned to Mayo as my research fellow in 1973 and 1974. Since the only book on the regulation of the venous system (edited by K. J. Franklin) dated from 1937, Vanhoutte and I summarized the current knowledge by writing *Veins and Their Control* in 1975.

In 1978 the Franqui Foundation in Brussels offered me an International Franqui Chair, which permitted me three months at the medical school of the University of Antwerp. Vanhoutte was then head of the pharmacology laboratory and professor of pharmacology and physiology there. I presented twelve lectures on issues in medical research. The award gave me the opportunity to collaborate with Vanhoutte on a book about the human cardiovascular system. Paul assigned me an office that overlooked a field. Just after my arrival, a mare kept in the field gave birth to a foal. We challenged ourselves to complete our book before the youngster reached maturity. Our textbook for medical students and young researchers was published in English in 1979 as *The Human Cardiovascular System: Facts and Concepts* and was eventually translated into Japanese among other languages.

In November 1979 I addressed the Royal Flemish Academy of Medicine in Brussels at the Paleis der Academien for an International Franqui Colloquium commemorating the academy's sesquicentennial. I spoke at the invitation of Albert Lacquet, an alumnus of the Mayo Graduate School of Medicine, who was the president of Koninklijke Academie voor Geneeskunde van België and head of surgery at the medical school of the University of Louvain (Leuven). Isodore Leusen, another Distinguished Mayo Alumnus who also was a member of the academy, was at the time chair of the Department of Physiology at the University of Ghent (Gent). ("Ghent" and "Louvain" reflect the spelling of the French-speaking majority in Belgium; in Flanders, the minority Flemish spell the words "Gent" and "Leuven.") My charge was to review the history of medical research in Belgium, where people speak Flemish *or* French. My speech was in English, my slides in Flemish! The address must have been well received because Lacquet informed me in May 1982 that I had been elected as a foreign member of the Royal Flemish Academy of Medicine.

The tensions between the Flemish-speaking minority and French-speaking majority in Belgium are deep and long-standing, as evidenced by an incident involving Paul Vanhoutte. In 1973, he became head of the pathophysiology laboratory at the University of Antwerp's medical school. There he presented (in Flemish) the results of his research for his doctorate, which he had conducted at Mayo. Some examiners at the oral defense of his thesis knew that when he had lived in Gent (Ghent) he had spoken French with his family at home—a socially unacceptable practice in Flanders. They informed him that while the science was excellent, his Flemish needed improvement. He would have to rewrite his dissertation before he could receive the degree. He did, but you can imagine how Vanhoutte, a native of Flanders, reacted!

Vanhoutte worked at Mayo a third time, from 1981 to 1989, as a consultant in the Department of Physiology and Biophysics with a joint appointment in the Department of Cardiovascular Medicine. He had organized a symposium on mechanisms of vasodilation in Wilrijk, Belgium, in 1977, which has since continued at various medical centers, always with international speakers. Vanhoutte arranged to have the 1986 meeting at the Mayo Clinic in my honor. That same year he established the John T. Shepherd Lecture for the Mechanisms of Vasodilation Symposia. I had the pleasure of attending the 2001 symposium and introducing my longtime friend, François M. Abboud of the University of Iowa College of Medicine, who is internationally known for his analyses of the complexity of the reflexes regulating the heart and circulation.

Richard Alan Cohen, another Distinguished Mayo Alumnus, also played a major role in organizing and conducting the 2001 symposium. He joined Paul Vanhoutte and me as a research fellow in 1981; he stayed on another year as an assistant professor of physiology and research associate. Cohen was from the vascular medicine section at Boston University Hospital and an assistant professor at the Boston University School of Medicine. He demonstrated his skills as an original investigator by examining the role of the endothelium in modulating the response of coronary arteries in dogs to different stimuli and how the action of the nerves supplying the arteries may be modified by events at their junction with the arteries. Cohen continued his studies after returning to Boston, further helping to demonstrate the dysfunction of the vascular endothelium in diabetes mellitus. He is now the Jay and Louise Coffman Professor of Vascular Medicine at the Boston University School of Medicine and director of the Vascular Biology Unit at Boston Medical Center.

During my later years at Mayo, I enjoyed doing research with two younger colleagues, Michael Joyner and Zvonimir S. Katusic. Our work dated back to my days at Queen's University, when Henry Barcroft first got me interested in research of the heart and circulation. He demonstrated during World War II that the decrease in arterial blood pressure that characterizes fainting is not caused by the sudden slowing of the heart, as commonly assumed, but by the marked dilation of small arteries (arterioles) in skeletal muscles. Since there are many such muscles, with many local and nervous factors continually adjusting the caliber of the arterioles, they play an important role in regulating arterial blood pressure. A change in the nerve supply to the muscle blood vessels—either an abrupt decrease in the activity of the nerves adjusting the degree of constriction of these vessels or an abrupt increase in activity causing them to dilate—could be the culprit.

Many years later, in 1987, Michael Joyner, a clinician-investigator in Mayo's Department of Anesthesiology, collaborated with me in the study of how these nerves adjust blood flow to skeletal muscles in normal subjects during gravitational stress. But we did not discover what causes dilation in muscles during fainting. We still have much to learn of the mechanisms that govern how humans respond to stress in normal and abnormal circumstances.

Four years earlier, Zvonimir Katusic, a 1977 medical graduate of the University of Belgrade, became a research fellow in Mayo's Department of Physiology and Biophysics in 1983. I proposed that he apply for a visiting fellowship, a training program I had established some years before. Thus, Katusic spent the year with Solomon H. Snyder at Johns Hopkins University Medical School in Baltimore. Snyder was a cowinner of the Wolf Prize in Medicine in 1982 for his work in developing ways to label the many receptors on which various neurotransmitters act. After returning to Mayo, Katusic has contributed to genetic analysis and its potential therapy in the vascular diseases, especially those involving the circulation to the brain.

All of my research fellows have pursued successful careers, but I have been a major beneficiary. In recognition of my role in training those who are now contributing to academic medicine, I have received several honorary degrees and memberships. After his Mayo fellowship, for example, Ettore Ambrosioni returned to the University of Bologna in Italy, where he became a professor of clinical medicine. Upon his recommendation, the university awarded me a *laurea honoris causa* in medicine in 1984. In 1985 the University of Ghent in Belgium awarded me a *diploma ad honores van doctor in de Geneeskunde.* In 1982 I received an honorary membership in the Irish Cardiac Society and became a member, in 1986, of the International Union of Angiology and, in 1996, the Worldwide Hungarian Medical Academy. My alma mater, Queen's University of Belfast, awarded me an honorary doctorate of science in 1979. (Another Irishman honored at the same time was celebrated flautist James Galway.)

visiting scientists and a hijacking

Two colleagues who worked with me at Mayo as visiting scientists deserve special mention. Yeouda Edoute joined Paul Vanhoutte and me at Mayo in 1985 to examine how certain local chemical changes inhibited the activity of the nerves that regulate the caliber of blood vessels in dogs. Edoute also investigated abnormalities in the blood supply to isolated hearts of rats with high blood pressure. A 1975 graduate of Hebrew University's Hadassah Medical School for his thesis on cardiac pacing in heart disease, Edoute had worked in the Department of Physiology and Medical Biochemistry at the University of Stellenbosch Medical School in Cape Town, South Africa. There he earned a doctorate in 1980 for his thesis on the ultrastructure and function in the oxygen-deprived rat heart. He lectured in the physiology of the heart at the Faculty of Medicine's Department of Physiology at the Technion in Haifa from 1980 until 1984. After his return to Haifa, Edoute joined the Rambam Medical Center as a cardiologist and internist, continued his research, and published additional scientific papers. Later, he became Rambam's head of Internal Medicine, Department C, and professor of medicine.

Two decades earlier, I worked with another distinguished international scientist, Israeli physiologist Shlomo (Moni) Samueloff of Hebrew University's Hadassah Medical School in Jerusalem. A Bulgarian by birth, Samueloff immigrated to Israel in 1949. He joined Norman Browse and me as a visiting scientist in 1964 in an additional study of the reflexes that regulate the caliber of the limb veins.

A few years after he returned to Israel following his fellowship at Mayo, Samueloff found himself in the hands of terrorists and at the center of international politics. He was returning to Israel after a visit in London with British scientists, including Browse, to discuss his research when his TWA flight was hijacked August 29, 1969, by Syrians and diverted from Tel Aviv to Damascus. In Damascus, the Syrians detained four Israeli women and two Israeli men, one of them Samueloff, before releasing the airliner and the rest of its passengers. The women were released after a day, but the men remained imprisoned.

Samueloff's wife, Naomi, contacted Browse in London, who in turn cabled me in Rochester: "Samueloff in prison Damascus. Can you get Mayo Trustees to release a Mayo Alumnus?" I replied at once that we had contacted Congressman Al Quie (who represented southeast Minnesota), the U.S. State Department, U.N. Secretary-General U Thant, and the Italian embassy in Damascus, since there was no U.S. embassy in Syria. We also contacted top officials of Damascus University Medical School.

Nearly two weeks after the hijacking, on September 11, Piero Ferraboschi of the Italian diplomatic staff in Damascus informed me that his government's ambassador in Syria had assured him "that every way to have Prof. Samueloff released is being explored. At the same time our ambassador in Damascus hinted that perhaps some pressure from national or international medical associations could find the Syrian authorities receptive and be of help in freeing Prof. Samueloff."

Samueloff's colleagues in England had already begun to apply pressure for his release, including an appeal to the director general of the World Health

Organization, which warned that "the spread of hijacking could imperil not merely the individuals directly but also the developing international collaboration in healthcare and medical research, and hence the very existence of WHO." Despite all efforts, the Syrians continued to hold Samueloff and his companion, releasing them only after an exchange of prisoners with Israel ninety-nine days after the hijacking.

"The overwhelming welcome of the many friends, organizations, and unknown people at home has started to calm down," Moni Samueloff wrote to me shortly after his return to Jerusalem. "I have finally the possibility to write the personal letters, which I have kept so long in my heart. From the copies of correspondence, which I have received since my return, I see that I am indefinitely obliged to you, John, for your effort to achieve my release."

He continued: "At the end of the first month, I received books from home brought to me by the Red Cross Representative. To see the Red Cross Representative for us, the prisoners, was just like a sunray in the dark. Together with the books received at first was also the *Mayo Alumnus* issue. It was such a good feeling to recall in the prison the peaceful and nice atmosphere of Rochester."

The dean of the medical faculty at Hebrew University in Jerusalem, Jonathan Magnes, also wrote to me that he was convinced that the support of Samueloff's international colleagues "was of the utmost importance in creating public opinion and, through this, in influencing the attitude of the Syrian authorities to the prisoners. Moreover, your moral support was of great value to Prof. Samueloff's family and colleagues." Diplomat Uri Oren dedicated his 1970 book *99 Days in Damascus* to the Samueloff family, with profound gratitude to those who participated in the efforts to free the two men imprisoned in Damascus.

scientific papers and books

The biomedical information gained through my studies over the years with all these research fellows and associates has been published in 236 peer-reviewed papers in twenty-nine scientific journals, as well as in scores of abstracts and eight books I have written and edited.

How proud I was when I submitted my first research paper for publication! That was in 1948, after approval of my thesis for a master's degree in surgery at Queen's University of Belfast. I sent my paper to *Clinical Science,* a distinguished academic medical journal in Great Britain. I soon received a note from George Pickering, the journal's editor, who asked me to come to his office the next time I was in London. Pickering was then professor of medicine at St. Mary's Hospital in London. Later he became Regius Professor of Medicine at Oxford University and was knighted by Queen Elizabeth.

I accepted Pickering's invitation and arrived as he was changing into his tuxedo for a formal dinner. "You start at the beginning and tell me what you want to say," he said as he continued dressing. As I told him my ideas, he would say, "Write this down," and so we continued to the end. "Now write that up and I will publish it," said Pickering, now dressed. As he left the room he added, "Next time you write a paper, put it in a drawer for a couple of weeks, then reread it before submitting it to a journal." This was a lesson I never forgot. I acknowledged Pickering for "rewriting my first paper" in my first medical book, *Physiology of the Circulation in Human Limbs in Health and Disease,* published in 1963.

That first paper, published in 1950, addressed research I conducted alone, but subsequent papers involved studies in which I was but one of several investigators. The publication of choice for those of us in the physiology department at Queen's was the prestigious *Journal of Physiology.* Unlike others, the *Journal of Physiology* listed names on the papers it published in alphabetical order. Supposedly, you would have a harder time achieving success if the first letter of your surname wasn't near the beginning or the end of the alphabet! During my early career in the British Isles, I often collaborated with younger colleagues whose names began with the letters R and W. My name always appeared between theirs. After my arrival at Mayo, only the determined efforts of a distinguished colleague convinced those responsible for promotions and research grants that I was indeed capable of independent investigation!

The order in which authors' names appear on a paper is indeed an important matter. The usual practice is to list first the prime mover in the conduct of the study, including preparation of the paper for publication. The last named usually is the first author's preceptor, commonly named as the senior author. Those in between have made varying contributions. As far as possible, I adopted the principle that a research fellow playing the key role in an experiment would be the sole author of a paper. Hence, none could doubt the credit was his.

Today, with multiple-choice questions being the prime method for testing student knowledge, it is not surprising that much of what is written for publication is mere verbiage. I have also noticed, as computer usage has matured, a tendency to confuse data with ideas and to mistake information for knowledge. Sir George Pickering insisted there be one minimum standard for degrees, namely that recipients be able to express themselves lucidly and grammatically in at least one language, preferably their own. Based on his teaching and my many years of training younger medical postgraduates, I insisted that, before they commenced a project, my research fellows write an introduction for the paper and answer the question: Why was the research project important? This exercise often exposed illiteracies, ambiguities, and illogicalities, which they would then have to address.

Since research teaches constructive thinking, even for those who do not continue research, each student in the Mayo Medical School must undertake a research project and write a paper. I consider research a valuable experience in creativity for anyone in residency training, even those planning careers in clinical medicine.

My contributions to scientific journals include membership on several editorial boards, a time-consuming but nevertheless important professional responsibility. I have served on the editorial boards of the *American Heart Journal, American Journal of Physiology, Cardiovascular Research, Circulation, Circulation Research, Clinical Autonomic Research, Hypertension, International Angiology, Journal of the Autonomic Nervous System,* and *Microvascular Research and Vascular Medicine.* I was also chief editor from 1988 to 1994 of the journal *News in Physiological Sciences.*

Sir Thomas Lewis, the English cardiologist who pioneered electrocardiography, played a key role in establishing clinical investigation as a scientific medical discipline. Lewis started the journal *Heart* (since 1933 known as *Clinical Science*) to encourage research on clinical problems. He taught by his example that when sufficient new data is available in a particular field of medicine, especially one to which you have contributed, a monograph or book analyzing the current state of knowledge is in order.

I took Lewis at his word and published eight books between 1963 and 1996, four of them with former research fellows at Mayo as coauthors. These were *Cardiac Function in Health and Disease* (1968) with Robert J. Marshall, also translated into Russian; *Veins and Their Control* (1975) and *The Human Cardiovascular System – Facts and Concepts* (1979), both with Paul M. Vanhoutte; and *Vascular Diseases in the Limbs: Mechanisms and Principles of Treatment* (1993) with Denis L. Clement. The scientific contributions of the fellows with whom I collaborated provided the main stimulus for all these books.

Along with François M. Abboud of the University of Iowa Medical School, I edited a handbook of physiology, *Peripheral Circulation and Organ Blood Flow.* Our 1983 volume was part of a continuing series of handbooks established by the American Physiological Society to provide scholarly, comprehensive, and critical analyses of specific organ systems. Each of these handbooks is massive—ours had a total of 1,063 pages—and includes contributions from multiple experts. Once you have accomplished such a project, you vow never to repeat the process! But this was not to be. In 1990 the American Physiological Society decided to produce a handbook titled *The Physiology of Exercise,* providing an in-depth analysis of regulatory mechanisms, including the signals responsible for the close matching of motor, cardiovascular, respiratory, and metabolic control during exercise. Unsolved problems concerning the origin of these signals have captured the imagination of investigators for more than a century. Finding no takers to commit themselves to this formidable and somewhat controversial task, I succumbed to an overpowering appeal to undertake the project, this time with Loring B. Rowell, an expert on exercise at the University of Washington. Our endeavor took five years but resulted in a single volume of 1,210 pages, with contributions from multiple experts, published in 1996.

When I achieved emeritus status at Mayo in 1990, I had more time to focus on several enjoyable aspects of my research. This included editing the book *Nervous Control of the Heart: The Human Cardiovascular System – Facts and Concepts* (1996) with Stephen F. Vatner, then at Harvard Medical School. Our book, published in English, was translated into Japanese.

funding research at Mayo

I served as chair of Mayo's Department of Physiology and Biophysics from 1966 to 1974, and in 1990 received the Distinguished Achievement Award from the U.S. Association of Chairmen of Departments of Physiology. My years as department chair coincided with my appointment in 1969 as the Mayo Clinic's first director for research, a position I held until 1977, as well as with my appointment as chair of the Institutional Research Committee. That I was also a member of the Mayo board of governors (from 1966 to 1980) and of the Mayo Foundation board of trustees (from 1969 to 1981) helped me to do my job as chair of the Institutional Research Committee.

Before 1959, the year that the Institutional Research Committee was created, a research administrative committee of Mayo's board of governors oversaw research. Earnings from the clinic's medical practice back then were sufficient to support both education and research, and there was no critical analysis of the quality of the various research programs.

Until 1957, when Mayo changed its policy and first applied for outside funds for research, a Mayo scientist could conduct research without thought of what he or she must accomplish to ensure the work's support by government funds. This made for easy interaction between investigators and clinicians. Research, like education, was seen as a component inseparable from medical practice. The principle was that physicians and scientists must integrate their efforts to achieve advances in medical practice.

When Senator Homer T. Bone of Washington urged Will Mayo in the 1930s to apply for federal funds for research, the physician refused. Mayo was adamantly opposed to having the government involved in the clinic's affairs. He was no less resistant to outside money from private sources. When a prominent and wealthy patient—one of the six Anderson brothers from Texas who came to Mayo for medical care in the late 1940s—asked whether the clinic could use extra money for cancer research, the answer was an emphatic no. (The brothers later founded the M. D. Anderson Cancer Hospital in Houston.)

The years after World War II saw a dramatic increase in medical research, and a consensus began to emerge in the 1950s that Mayo could not sustain its long-standing policy against accepting outside funds. At last, in 1957, the clinic changed its policy: Mayo would henceforth seek and accept extramural funding for research from both the public and private sectors. Patients would be assured their medical and surgical fees were not inflated to support education and research. Neither would the clinical staff be called on to support these activities beyond reason.

The major source of funding for biomedical research in the United States is the National Institutes of Health, a federal agency within the Public Health Service. The NIH encompasses twenty-seven institutes and centers, occupies more than three hundred acres in Bethesda, Maryland, and employs eighteen thousand people. Alexander Albert, an endocrinologist, applied for and received Mayo's first NIH research grant to study thyroid disease and disorders of the pituitary gland.

"The internist and the surgeon must join with the laboratory scientists to lead medicine to greater heights," Will Mayo once noted. "Union of these forces will lengthen by many years the span of human life." True to its mission, the Mayo Clinic continues to provide high-quality, compassionate patient care at a reasonable cost through a physician-led team of diverse people working together in clinical practice, education, and research in a unified multicampus system.

The year after I joined the board of governors, 1967, was significant for the Mayo Clinic, for the board then addressed the disproportion between income and the rising costs of operations. Spending for research had increased from 48 percent of total costs in 1964 to 65 percent in 1967. The board asked me to select a task force to review research projects in progress with the goal of controlling expenditures and ensuring that institutional costs were proportioned to institutional objectives.

The assignment, not strictly a financial matter, included scientific and social challenges. Thus, my first priority was to assemble a group of Mayo staff members knowledgeable about the research programs undertaken. The group would decide which of these research programs deserved continuing support and then develop principles for the support of future research programs.

Our report to the governors the following year became known as "the Blue Book" because it was bound in a blue cover. Mayo then had a staff of 478, of whom 119 were engaged in research of some kind. We found that 40 percent would be unable ever to obtain outside financial support. Our task force recommended primary criteria for researchers: that only competent investigators should continue in research; that all researchers must be capable of independent investigation and of obtaining extramural funds; that clinical groups should form clinical research sections whenever possible, and that members of basic medical sciences departments should have joint appointments with clinical disciplines; and last, that a budgetary system should be developed to allocate research funds.

The task force also recommended closing some programs, but our recommendations did not necessarily decide the matter. Objecting to our decision to close his laboratory, for example, one staff member continued his research until I finally had to put a lock on the door. We did better when we decided to close a section that had run its course. The report recommended giving priority to research in laboratory medicine, pharmacology, clinical pharmacology, experimental oncology, bioengineering, and medical biochemistry. It also recommended that Mayo continue development of a clinical research unit at Saint Marys Hospital.

Mayo implemented all of our recommendations, eventually coming more and more to depend on funds secured through the development program established in 1969. The 1957 decision to secure extramural funding for research meant that all of us who had received Mayo funds for research now had to secure outside funding. Such funding must pay the salaries of research fellows (unless their own institutions or countries would pay them), the cost of technical assistance, and the prorated salary of the staff scientist heading the program, according to the amount of time he or she is involved.

Mayo must compete with every other applicant in the United States who has applied for financial support to the NIH, the major funder of research. Depending on the size of the NIH budget approved by Congress, an investigator may have to submit applications repeatedly before receiving funds. (Someone has observed that research is the absence of prejudice backed by the presence of money. Another wit has noted that all great discoveries are made by mistake, and the greater the funding, the longer it takes to make the mistake!)

Congress often influences the sort of research that gets funded, sometimes directing the NIH to make grants in one area or another. During one period, politics played such a prominent role in funding that we scientists sniffed at the "Disease of the Month Club." Others in Congress have questioned, even ridiculed, research programs funded by the NIH. Senator William Proxmire of Wisconsin, for example, singled out projects he considered silly or irrelevant with his Golden Fleece Awards. These more often than not reflected Proxmire's misguided judgments. One study that he named, on "variations in the color of butterfly wings," led to the discovery of the Rh factor in human blood. Another on "the nerve fiber of the squid" helped us understand how nerves function and led to much of what we know about the origins of irregular heart rhythms.

creating the Pharmacology Department

As Mayo's first director for research, I recognized a need for a pharmacology department. (Departments were previously called sections.) Pharmacology is a key link between basic medical science and clinical medicine; as such, it is essential in translating basic advances and understanding into patient care. Clinical pharmacology helps us understand how drugs act and which are suitable for different patients. The coming age of pharmacogenetics may make it possible for us provide a patient with a specific treatment for his or her malady. With the support of Richard Reitemeier, chair of the Department of Medicine, the board of governors supported my recommendation and provided $6 million to establish the Department of Pharmacology over a period of several years.

Organizing the new department took more than the approval of the Mayo governors. Because the clinic was then part of the Graduate School of Medicine of the University of Minnesota, I also consulted the chair of the university's Department of Pharmacology as a courtesy.

Fortunately for Mayo, the medical school at Harvard University was just then engaged in an extensive review of its own outstanding pharmacology department. In the absence of definite plans, another department had already seized some of its research space, and some of its brightest stars had begun to look elsewhere. One of these dynamic younger Harvard scientists was John Blinks, who accepted our invitation to lead the new Department of Pharmacology at Mayo. His joining the staff in 1967 resulted in other outstanding appointments to the new venture.

Based on the "Blue Book" recommendation, we had closed the Section of Biophysics and allocated its limited space in the Medical Sciences Building to the pharmacology department. I assured Blinks that we intended to allocate more suitable space for the new department in a planned research building: the Guggenheim Building. We were also planning a diagnostic laboratory building: the Hilton Building. A site for these two proposed buildings was available just south of the Mayo and Plummer Buildings. (Another candidate clearly thought this was just a recruitment ploy. After the new department had settled in the new building, he called to ask for a return visit. He wanted to check on whether I had told him the truth about the new research buildings!)

As director for research, my practice was to anticipate and refer requests for space for research programs—always a challenge—to a small subcommittee for recommendations. For instance, before allocating the area for construction of the Guggenheim and Hilton Buildings, I asked Saint Marys Hospital administrators whether they might want the same space for future expansion. They decided that Saint Marys would continue to build on the hospital's ample existing site. On another occasion, when John Kirklin transferred his open-heart surgery program from Rochester Methodist Hospital to Saint Marys, he sought an extra room near the operating room for processing data on his patients and writing papers. Although I sent his request at once to the subcommittee, the brilliant, dynamic Kirklin had little patience for protracted committee discussions and instead went directly to the Sisters of Saint Francis, who run Saint Marys Hospital, and at once obtained the room he required. I suspect Kirklin would have appreciated Lord Milverton's statement: "The ideal committee is one with me as chairman and the other two members in bed with flu."

the Guggenheim and Hilton Buildings

In the years following Mayo's decision to accept outside funds, the clinic received generous gifts, many from wealthy patients who had benefited from care at Mayo. Two such gifts came from Edmond Guggenheim and Conrad N. Hilton and made it possible in 1974 for Mayo to open the two adjacent research buildings that bear their names.

Edmond Guggenheim was the grandson of Meyer Guggenheim, a Swiss-born Jewish immigrant to America in 1848. Meyer Guggenheim built a successful business importing lace but greatly increased his fortune after investing in Colorado silver mines in 1881. His family business, the American Smelting and Refining Company, eventually expanded into copper and nitrates in Colorado, Mexico, Alaska, Chile, and other places around the world. Five of Meyer's seven sons worked in the family business. Four of them gave away hundreds of millions of dollars through their philanthropic foundations to support their various interests, including university-based aeronautic institutes, the New York Botanical Gardens, and various Guggenheim Museums around the world.

After the death of his father in 1939, Edmond Guggenheim took over the leadership of his family's Murry and Leonie Guggenheim Foundation. In the late 1960s, near the end of his life, he closed out the foundation to distribute its assets among several institutions. It was just at that time that my colleague Emmerson Ward, a rheumatologist who was then chair of Mayo's board of governors, had a fortuitous conversation with Guggenheim. When Guggenheim asked how Mayo would use a substantial grant, the clinic responded with a proposal for financial support of a new research building.

Within weeks Mayo received from Guggenheim a gift of nearly $9 million, which covered about half the anticipated cost of construction. Since that was the principle we had established for naming buildings, the new twelve-story facility became the Guggenheim Building for Research and Education in the Life Sciences. The Guggenheim Building opened in 1974 and expanded in 1990 to the full twenty floors of its design. The addition more than doubled the space available for Mayo research departments.

The Guggenheim Building marked a major advance in Mayo's research potential. In its complementary role as an educational facility, the building provides resources for the medical school and the postdoctoral programs of the graduate school. Among educational facilities in the building are three amphitheater-style lecture halls and eight seminar rooms, four of them equipped with facilities for laboratory exercises and demonstrations.

On the main floor are plaques recognizing other major Mayo benefactors, including Robert Anderson, chair of Rockwell International, and Ruth and Bruce Rappaport, chair of Inter Maritime Bank. Mayo's two Nobel laureates, Edward C. Kendall and Phillip S. Hench, are also honored with plaques. (Kendall joined Mayo in 1914 as the clinic's first scientist dedicated to biochemical research. Hench joined Mayo as a rheumatologist in 1926. Kendall and Hench received the Nobel Prize in physiology or medicine in 1950 for discoveries relating to the hormones of the adrenal cortex, Kendall for his discovery of cortisone and Hench for demonstrating its effectiveness in rheumatic diseases.)

After construction on the Guggenheim Building was under way, the architects found that the space available for offices for staff was less than the requirement. So these offices turned out to be not quite as large as we had hoped. As director for research, I received the complaints, mostly about noise from adjoining offices. The chief architect recommended we install a machine to mask sounds from other offices with "white noise." In the end, he solved the problem by increasing the insulation between offices.

Mayo also opened in 1974 the Hilton Building for Laboratory Medicine, which came about through the generosity of Conrad N. Hilton, founder of the international hotel corporation bearing his name. Until then, Mayo's clinical diagnostic laboratories were physically separate, but our policy of buying property and land in downtown Rochester adjacent to the Mayo campus meant we had space available to integrate the diagnostic laboratories in one building. While there were arguments against doing so, I favored integrating our laboratories in a new building and connecting them with our research facilities in the Guggenheim Building. That would permit close interaction between researchers and those who were designing and developing new tests and procedures.

When Hilton indicated he would consider a major gift to Mayo, the board of governors met with him to describe the proposed building. We were looking for a gift of $10 million toward the overall cost of the building. Hilton asked for a detailed proposal, which we sent at once. A few weeks later we received a letter from the Conrad N. Hilton Foundation confirming a ten-year, $10 million pledge, with a $1 million check for the initial payment. A plaque in the building's entrance acknowledges Hilton's generous philanthropy "to aid the sick through education, research, and clinical studies in

Laboratory Medicine." Beside the plaque is a bust of Conrad Hilton, completed in 1972 by the sculptor Charles Eugene Gagnon.

To design and construct both the Guggenheim and Hilton Buildings, the board of governors selected the Ellerbe Company, a Minnesota firm with a long association with the Mayo Clinic. Ellerbe had designed and built the 1914 red-brick building, the 1928 Plummer Building, the 1952 Medical Sciences Building, and the 1957 Mayo Building. During planning for the new buildings, I hoped aloud that the architects might be able to solve an environmental problem: tall buildings cause the velocity of the wind to increase. For patients coming out of such a building, sometimes in wheelchairs, the wind can be bitterly uncomfortable. Alas, there is yet no solution.

In the many years of my involvement with medical research at Mayo, I have learned that nothing succeeds in moving research ahead as much as when clinical colleagues are our advocates. To the extent that researchers interact effectively with clinical colleagues, not as servants or technicians but as independent investigators undertaking studies with important biomedical implications, so our research prospers. Continuing close alliance and interplay between physicians, clinician-investigators, and basic scientists results in advances for the better care of our patients that is the true spirit of Mayo.

Of special importance is the role of the clinician-investigator, knowledgeable in medical practice and skilled in research. The clinician-investigator can interpret information obtained in the laboratory for the care of the patient and take patient problems to the laboratory. Former NIH director James Wyngaarden has described the clinician-investigator as an endangered species because of the great challenge of being both a capable medical practitioner and a competitive original investigator. Perhaps, but my experience shows that the clinician-investigator is not (as one wit suggested) a half-trained scientist and a half-baked clinician. Instead, the clinician-investigator is a person with exceptional talents and abilities. In the new world of genetic analysis and therapy particularly, the clinician-investigator will fill a key role in translating the language and discoveries of the molecular biologists to the clinicians and the key medical problems of the physicians to the biologists. I believe clinician-investigators are essential to advance the coming new era in medicine.

Mayo research branches out

The Mayo Clinic was once synonymous with Rochester, Minnesota. With the addition in the 1980s of two major Mayo centers in Jacksonville, Florida, and Scottsdale, Arizona, the board of governors decided that both new clinics would follow the Rochester model. That meant that the two centers would establish their own education and research programs. Scientists at all three Mayo centers focus on genetic research in particular, as we can develop specific gene therapies to cure and prevent diseases once we have determined their genetic basis. Analysis of the human genome makes this an exciting time, and Mayo scientists adding to our knowledge in this complex but vital area at Rochester, Jacksonville, and Scottsdale are skilled and dedicated.

At Scottsdale, medical research takes place in nine laboratories at the Samuel C. Johnson Medical Research Building, opened in November 1993 and named for the former chair of Mayo's board of trustees who provided funds for the building. Johnson was the fourth generation of his family to head the Johnson Wax firm, headquartered in Racine, Wisconsin.

At Jacksonville, the Davis School of Medical Sciences supports Mayo programs in education and research. Established in 1995, the school represents a major philanthropic commitment by the Davis family, founders of Winn-Dixie, one of the largest supermarket chains in the United States, to ensure Mayo's leadership in the new century. The Davis family's overall goal is to bring improved health care to communities where they and their associates live and work. James E. Davis in 1948 was the first member of his family to be a patient at Mayo. Robert, Wayne, Charles, and Dano Davis (now chair and CEO of Winn-Dixie Stores) represent the second generation of Davis family philanthropy to Mayo. To recognize this enduring friendship, Mayo commissioned a wall display in front of the Davis School of Medical Sciences.

With the help of an invocation by the Reverend Billy Graham, Mayo dedicated the John H. and Jennie D. Birdsall Medical Research Building in Jacksonville in October 1993. Respected business leaders in Palm Beach, Florida (John founded the construction company that bears his name and its shipping subsidiary), the Birdsalls have been generous supporters of Alzheimer's and related dementia research programs.

(In the long tradition of medicine, diseases have been named for their discoverer, with no indication of their specific nature. Thus, Alzheimer's disease is named for the German urologist Alois Alzheimer, Parkinson's for the English physician James Parkinson. The practice of naming diseases prompted S. J. Perelman's wry comment, "I've got Bright's disease, and he's got mine.")

At Mayo Jacksonville's Institute of Neurodegenerative Diseases, research focuses on diseases such as Alzheimer's, Parkinson's, and ALS (amyotrophic lateral sclerosis, or Lou Gehrig's disease). In 2000 a Jacksonville neurobiologist, Michael Hutton, was a co-recipient of the Potamkin Award of the American Academy of Neurobiologists for research in Pick's, Alzheimer's, and related diseases.

William Summerskill

In my long career at the Mayo Clinic, I have made many dear friends among distinguished colleagues. One was William Summerskill, a Mayo consultant, director of the gastroenterology unit, and professor and vice chair of the Department of Medicine.

A graduate of Oxford University Medical School who had done postgraduate training at Harvard University Medical School, Summerskill became an acknowledged international leader in diseases of the liver. At Mayo he established a renowned group to study diseases of the gastrointestinal system and made numerous contributions to research, for which he received a doctorate of science from Oxford. Upon learning of my British education and honorary degrees, he nominated me as an honorary fellow of the Royal College of Physicians of London. I was elected FRCP in 1977.

Bill Summerskill was also a neighbor, and he often invited Helen and me to cruise along the Mississippi River on his boat with him and his wife, Barbara. We had many opportunities to discuss important issues, particularly when he was a member of the Mayo Research Committee at the time I was chair. After completing my assignment as director for research, I became director for education in 1977. Bill and Barbara held a dinner in their home to honor me and others who had served on the research committee. He gave me that evening a presentation volume recalling our having taken our state medical board examinations together twenty years earlier. The memento also highlighted the achievements of the research committee in establishing the Department of Immunology and instituting other changes at Mayo.

Nominated to be my successor as director for research, Summerskill was also considering another academic opportunity in California. Before he could make a choice, however, he died suddenly on March 12, 1977. Not long before his death, Bill displayed what was to me a new talent as a poet. He wrote some verse to mark the end of my term as director for research. At his memorial service, I quoted the last verse of his little poem, changing but one word, to honor him: "Whatever deeds the man has rendered, / The person matters in the end / And as such, Bill, I gladly salute you, / Neighbor, counselor, and friend."

Having completed my tenure as Mayo's director of research in 1977, I continued my studies on the human cardiovascular system in the clinic's physiology department for many more years. Equally exciting were the opportunities I was given to make research contributions beyond the Mayo Clinic, at venues as varied as the American Heart Association, the National Institutes of Health—even NASA.

3

NASA and beyond

My ongoing pursuits in cardiovascular research in Mayo's physiology department eventually took me beyond the city of Rochester, Minnesota, and the clinic itself to collaborate in a variety of roles with colleagues at other institutions, often in other countries. Especially memorable was a trip in the 1980s to the Soviet Union as a member of the U.S. delegation of scientists who met with our Russian counterparts to discuss diseases of the heart and circulation.

My experiences as a Mayo Clinic administrator – eight years as director of research, eight years as chair of the department of physiology and biophysics – also served me well when in 1975 I became president of the American Heart Association. And my decades as an often-published medical scientist prepared me for a stint as a research fraud investigator in 1981 for the National Institutes of Health, which followed my earlier committee work on the cardiovascular system for that well-respected organization.

But of all my research opportunities beyond the Mayo Clinic, perhaps the most far-reaching – literally – began in 1965 when I joined the National Academy of Sciences' Committee on Space Biology and Medicine. That position, as well as my appointment to the academy's Space Science Board, allowed me to continue my work on arterial blood pressure and the cardiovascular effects of flight on humans. Ultimately, my work with the academy led to a plum assignment: my appointment to NASA's Life Sciences Advisory Committee, which gave me front-row exposure to our country's historic race into space against the Soviet Union and to America's extraordinary mission of landing the first man on the moon.

the new frontier of space

On October, 4, 1957, I listened with amazement to the news bulletin being broadcast over my car radio: the Soviets had launched *Sputnik,* the first artificial satellite, into space. Along with the rest of the world I learned that the 183-pound *Sputnik,* no bigger than a basketball, was circling Earth on its elliptical path every ninety-eight minutes. While I could not know that within a few years I would be engaged in the U.S. space program, I recognized the Soviets' achievement as a major event in the cold war between the democratic allies in the West and the Communist bloc in the East.

One month later, the Soviets launched *Sputnik 2,* which was not only much heavier (1,120 pounds) but also carried the first living being into space: a dog named Laika. The data that *Sputnik 2* sent back showed how Laika was adapting to space—critical information for the manned space missions already being planned. Because the Soviets had no way to return *Sputnik 2* to Earth safely, Laika was put to sleep, but the satellite itself remained in orbit 162 days.

The Soviets' successes caused the United States deep international embarrassment in the new space race. The humiliation increased when the first U.S. attempt two months after the launch of *Sputnik 1* ended with the rocket exploding on the launch pad. Of greater concern, the Soviets had raised fears that they might translate their advances into a military advantage that would tip the balance of power between East and West.

Germany sowed the seeds of the race for space during World War II when it developed the V-2 rocket, capable of flying at supersonic speeds. In the war's final weeks, the Americans and the Soviets both set their sights on capturing Germany's rocket laboratories, the stock of V-2 missiles, and the German scientists themselves. The Americans got V-2 inventor Wernher von Braun as well as some V-2 rockets, while the Soviets managed to snare other German scientists and blueprints for the V-2.

Under the direction of Sergei Pavlovich Korolev, the father of the Soviet Union's aerospace program, the Soviets advanced rapidly, and in 1959 they selected the first group of cosmonauts to begin training for space exploration. They accomplished their mission on April 12, 1961, when Yuri Gagarin became the first human in space aboard *Vostok 1.* During his historic 108-minute flight, Gagarin orbited Earth once and flew weightless for eighty-nine minutes between 112 and 155 miles above the planet. As *Vostok 1* returned to Earth through the atmosphere, Gagarin proved that people could withstand a G-force of at least 7.7.

The Soviets soon followed that epic manned mission with a second one, when Gherman Titov orbited the Earth seventeen times. On June 16, 1963, a little more than two years after Gagarin's first orbital flight, the Soviets sent the first woman into space. Valentina Vladimirovna Tereshkova orbited Earth in *Vostok 6* forty-five times, preceding the first U.S. woman in space, Sally Ride aboard the space shuttle *Challenger,* by twenty years.

Though plagued by technical problems—one of every three rockets exploded on the launch pad during the early days—the American space program put its first satellite, *Explorer 1,* into orbit on January 31, 1958. The thirty-pound satellite discovered the Van Allen radiation belts that surround the Earth. Eight months later the National Aeronautics and Space Administration—NASA—opened. On May 5, 1961, about three weeks after the Soviets' first manned flight, the United States sent its first astronaut, Alan Shepard, into space for a fifteen-minute suborbital flight in the *Liberty Bell 7* space capsule.

A perception that America had lost ground to the Soviet Union during Dwight Eisenhower's administration helped John F. Kennedy win the presidency in 1960. Just three weeks after Shepard's flight, Kennedy told Congress that "the nation should commit itself to achieving the goal, before this decade is out, of landing a man on the moon and returning him safely to earth. No single space project in this period will be more impressive to mankind or . . . be so difficult or expensive to accomplish."

After the failures and embarrassments of its early efforts, the U.S. space program was finally making progress, and the first American to orbit the Earth was John Glenn aboard *Mercury Friendship 7* on February 20, 1962. (In 1998, at the age of seventy-seven, Glenn became the oldest person in space aboard the shuttle *Discovery* after petitioning NASA to let him fly again to conduct space-based research on aging.)

Scientists were learning a great deal about the effects of space flight on the human body during the exciting years of NASA's Mercury, Gemini, and Apollo programs. A major medical concern with the first manned missions was the so-called cardiac deconditioning that occurred during the weightlessness of space flight. Because of the well-known pioneering studies on gravitational forces conducted at Mayo under the leadership of my first chief, Earl Wood, and my own research on the multiple complex factors regulating the heart and blood vessels, the National Academy of Sciences invited me in 1965 to join its Committee on Space Biology and Medicine, whose cardiovascular section I chaired from 1968 to 1974. In 1971 I joined NASA's Life

Sciences Advisory Committee for a two-year stint, and in 1973 became chair of the National Academy of Sciences' Committee on Space Medicine, part of its Space Science Board.

As the manned orbital flights continued, we kept an eye on President Kennedy's goal of putting a man on the moon before the end of the decade. But the Soviet Union had the same goal. Its *Luna 2,* the first probe to reach the moon, crash-landed in 1959, but its *Luna 9* landed safely in 1966. But just seven months after Frank Borman, James Lovell Jr., and William Anders orbited the moon in *Apollo 8,* Americans finally realized President Kennedy's vision. Together with Michael Collins, astronauts Neil Armstrong and Edwin (Buzz) Aldrin Jr. steered *Apollo 11* into orbit around the moon and on Sunday, July 20, 1969, landed the lunar module *Eagle* on the surface of the moon's Sea of Tranquility. As the world watched on television, Armstrong stepped onto the rock-strewn surface—"That's one small step for man, one giant leap for mankind"—followed eighteen minutes later by Aldrin.

As NASA prepared for the first lunar landing mission, our discussion at the National Academy of Sciences concerned the effects of heavy charged particles on the astronauts and the possibility that the men might bring back to Earth some unknown organism that would afflict humans. As a precaution, we quarantined the astronauts on their return from the moon—which, of course, proved quite unnecessary.

Even as NASA began to plan for routine space missions with the space shuttle program, the public's interest in space exploration seemed to dissipate following the lunar landing missions. Shortly after my appointment in 1973 to the Committee on Space Medicine of the National Academy's Space Science Board, William Proxmire of Wisconsin, as chair of a Senate appropriations subcommittee, wrote to inform me that he intended to recommend that the funds requested to continue development of the shuttle be dropped from the appropriations bill for fiscal year 1974. (NASA had awarded the primary shuttle contract in July 1972, nearly a decade before the first shuttle, *Columbia,* launched in 1981.) Anticipating an extensive debate about the topic when the bill reached the Senate floor, Proxmire said his subcommittee was anxious to have the views of prominent scientists who were familiar with the space program on whether the shuttle program should proceed.

A few days later, John Coleman, executive officer of the National Academy of Sciences, cautioned me to make it clear that my answers to Proxmire's questions reflected only *my* opinions, since the full Space Science Board "has not had benefit of full discussion of [the] matter." Consequently, I replied to Proxmire regarding "my personal views on the space shuttle," pointing out that as a new member I did not know whether the board had been asked about whether NASA should proceed with the shuttle. "Based on the assumption that the plans for the shuttle will proceed," I wrote, "I have regarded my primary role on the Space Science Board to determine how we can use the resources it provides for the total advancement of science and to maintain the leadership of the United States in the scientific exploration of space." Despite Proxmire's opposition, the full Senate approved funds for the space shuttle for fiscal year 1974.

I found that in the company of the distinguished physicists and astronomical scientists on the Space Science Board, my principal task was to support the NASA program of sending humans into space rather than relying solely on unmanned space vehicles. This was sometimes difficult, since most of my nonmedical colleagues believed that putting humans in space was more political than scientific. The key questions at this time concerned what weightlessness might do to the human cardiovascular system, how the astronauts would readjust to Earth's gravity, and how space travelers could be monitored so that we would know when to abort a mission.

In addition to attending meetings at the National Academy of Sciences in Washington, D.C., I also joined a group of medical scientists concerned with the cardiovascular system. We met regularly with a similar group of experts on the human respiratory system, including during one two-week session in 1965 at Wood's Hole on Cape Cod reviewing new information and advising NASA about future missions.

One question we considered was whether astronauts should continue to breathe pure oxygen on space missions, since this greatly heightened the danger of fire. We recommended that NASA change this practice and follow the example of the Soviets, who provided their cosmonauts with a normal atmosphere. NASA, however, rejected our recommendation—until a spark in the oxygen-filled cabin of *Apollo I* caused the fire that killed astronauts Virgil (Gus) Grissom, Edward White II, and Roger Chaffee on January 27, 1967. White had been the first American to walk in space. His historic twenty-one-minute walk occurred in 1965, the same year I began to participate in the space program. (By contrast, the hundredth space walk by an American occurred on February 14, 2001, and lasted five-and-a-half hours. That milestone came just two days before the space shuttle *Atlantis* undocked after four months from the international space station, leaving behind NASA's first permanent orbiting laboratory since the 1970s.)

As we contemplated long space flights and extended periods of time in space, the matter of how weightlessness affects the human body became increasingly important. Until we could learn from experience, our only relevant knowledge came from studies of the effects of prolonged bed rest on the cardiovascular-respiratory system. Such rest was thought to approximate the effect of weightlessness. A major goal of the manned space program was to check how the astronauts responded by gradually increasing the length of time in space. During space flights in the 1960s and 1970s, I often monitored medical events experienced by the astronauts and reported constantly by telemetry to NASA headquarters in Washington, D.C. With this information, I helped my NASA colleagues decide whether the mission should continue after each orbit of the Earth. When we were satisfied with an astronaut's physical status, we would say, "Let's give him another whirl."

We closely watched the medical condition of every astronaut. One of the original seven NASA astronauts, Donald (Deke) Slayton was grounded from space flights in the early 1960s because of an irregular heartbeat. Finally restored to full flight status in 1972, he piloted the joint American-Russian space flight mission in July 1975, *Apollo-Soyuz.* (Subsequently, in October 1976, while I was president of the American Heart Association, I presented Slayton with the AHA's "Heart of the Year" award at the Johnson Space Center in Houston.)

As a member of the National Academy of Sciences' Space Science Board, I attended many launches at Cape Kennedy. On one such occasion, I met King Hussein of Jordan, who was fascinated with developments in space exploration. Some years later, in 1998, Hussein began chemotherapy at the Mayo Clinic for non-Hodgkin's lymphoma. The disease was terminal, and he died in 1999 after a reign of forty-six years.

I was not the only one from Mayo associated with the U.S. space program. Bernard Harris, a Mayo fellow in internal medicine from 1982 to 1985, became an astronaut and in 1993 conducted a videoconference with Mayo staff from the space shuttle *Columbia.*

Shields Warren of the New England Deaconess Hospital in Boston, chair of the NASA Life Sciences Committee, wrote in 1974 to thank me for my "help and sound judgment [which] kept us heading in the right direction." In my reply, I predicted "continuing and appropriate interaction" between the Space Science Board and the Life Sciences Committee—two important groups—"for the betterment of our future space plans." I believe that has happened. My last association with the National Academy of Sciences was in 1993 as chair of the Academy-Research Council delegation to the International Physiological Sciences Congress and General Assembly in Glasgow, Scotland.

Also in 1974 NASA honored me with its Skylab Achievement Award. Years later I attended the thirtieth reunion of former members of the National Academy of Sciences' Space Science Board, where we were brought up to date on events in the U.S. space program. At the end of this occasion, the Space Science Board chair noted that in at least one respect nothing had changed in the past three decades: there was still no effective communication and interchange between the White House, NASA, and the National Academy!

It is my hope that, despite the tragedies of the 1986 *Challenger* and 2003 *Columbia* shuttle explosions, the U.S. space program will continue its important endeavors. Certainly the grand adventure in space has furthered medical research, but it has also taught us a vital lesson about peace among the multiplicity of diverse nations living on one planet. "Look at this little earth floating in this black sea that goes on forever," I commented in a 1989 interview with the *Rochester Post-Bulletin.* "That's all there is. Maybe that will teach the nations that if we're going to blow this up with bombs or destroy it with pollution, there isn't anywhere else to go."

I had in mind the classic photograph of Earth made by astronaut William Anders as *Apollo 8* orbited the moon in 1968. "We'd come nearly 240,000 miles to see the moon," Anders said of the photo, "and it was the Earth that was really worth looking at." Anders sent me a print of that famous photo. Among my other memorabilia marking my involvement with the U.S. space program is a virtually complete collection of space postage stamps, which I've added to my larger collection of the stamps of my adopted country, the United States.

American Heart Association

As a result of my research and my service on national committees relative to the cardiovascular system, the American Heart Association elected me its president in 1975. I had previously served as a member of the AHA's Research Committee from 1968 to 1973 (and chaired it from 1971 to 1972) and as chair of the AHA's Council on Circulation (from 1971 to 1973).

As president, I oversaw the AHA's move into new headquarters. The organization had been located for more than half a century in New York City, but by 1970 attracting and keeping staff was difficult and the existing location offered no room for expansion. The Burke Foundation had offered six acres of land on its campus in White Plains, New York, but the relocation committee rejected the offer, principally because of determined opposition to moving out of New York City. After conducting a nationwide search and considering thirty-six possibilities, a second relocation committee chose Dallas for its quality of life, including an international airport, several universities, and a medical school.

The AHA headquarters relocated in December 1975 to property owned by Presbyterian Hospital. (Texas oilman Toddy Lee Wynn helped arrange an offer for the AHA to lease the property from Presbyterian Hospital for ninety-nine years for only a dollar a year.) I was a member of the AHA board of directors in June 1972 when the committee proposed the move from New York City to Dallas. After endorsing the move, we paid the entire amount—$99! Board chair Richard D. Dotts and I presided over the dedication of the building on January 30, 1976. We framed the cancelled $99 check and hung it in a prominent place inside the building.

As part of my official duties as AHA president, I once gave an after-lunch address at a fund-raiser at the Doctor's Club in Houston emphasizing the importance of gaining new knowledge of heart disease through research. Jere Mitchell, president of the AHA's Texas affiliate, organized the event to raise money from wealthy Texans for support of cardiovascular research in that state. The Houston club was luxurious; my shoes almost disappeared in the thick carpets. Among the twenty or so guests was the flamboyant billionaire H. Ross Perot, who, after I finished my address, asked whether all the money he raised would be spent in Texas. When Mitchell told him it would be, Perot turned to his colleagues and said, "This is going to cost you $25,000 each, so write your checks now and let's get out of here." After all had done so, Perot told Mitchell, "Come with me in my plane, and I will leave you off in Dallas." The group disappeared, and I stood abandoned in the splendid surroundings!

I appeared at other such fund-raising events, including one at the headquarters of the AHA's Montana affiliate in Billings. Again, I gave an after-dinner talk on the importance of financial support for research pertinent to the cardiovascular diseases. As soon as I finished, the large audience departed, except for one man, who said, "You talk funny. Where do you come from?" When I told him I was from Rochester, Minnesota, he replied, "You don't talk like a Minnesotan. Where were you born?" When I told him I was born in Ireland, he asked me what happens if you cross an Irishman and a baboon. "You get a retarded baboon," he said as he departed, laughing heartily. Had he stayed, I might have told him about the man from Montana who made a trip to the west coast of Oregon and sat watching a new lighthouse. "It's no good," he told his colleagues when he returned home. "Lights flash and horns blow—but the fog still comes in!"

After my year as president of the American Heart Association, I received its Gold Heart Award in 1978. I then served from 1986 to 1990 on the AHA's Science Advisory Committee, which I chaired between 1986 and 1988. I was also on the association's Budget Committee (1988–1990) and chaired the Task Force on Vascular Medicine and Biology (1990–1992).

falsifying data in research

During the mid-1970s I became involved in the National Institutes of Health, first as a member of the project committee of its Heart and Lung Program (1973–1975) and then as a member of the National Heart, Lung, and Blood Institute's Hypertension Task Force in 1976. In December 1981 I joined a special National Institutes of Health panel of senior investigators experienced in cardiovascular research to deal with the issue of researchers who falsify their data. I considered the assignment so important that I removed my name from the list of candidates being considered for another NIH position, that of director of the National Heart, Lung, and Blood Institute. Recognizing the serious nature of our work, including the possibility of legal complications to our institutions as a consequence of our investigations, the NIH made the four of us on the panel federal employees during our six-month-long inquiry (since the federal government may not be sued).

Our task was to review the circumstances and events in a laboratory of a prestigious university medical school at which a young medical investigator had been reported for scientific misconduct. One of the investigator's colleagues had observed and reported his tampering with the data. A committee of senior scientists at the school had investigated the matter and concluded that a single episode of fraud had occurred.

Indeed, we found that the investigator had falsified data on *many* of the research projects in which he had been involved. As a consequence of our findings, the papers about his research already published in medical journals had to be formally withdrawn. While there was no evidence that any of the coauthors had fabricated data, they were understandably distraught. One coauthor said he did not even know his name was on the paper. In addition, we showed that the investigator had cheated in a joint study with investigators in three other prestigious university medical schools, also supported by the NIH. Our conclusions encouraged others to investigate the behavior of the perpetrator in the research published from his prior institution. Again, he was shown to have falsified data. The papers based on that earlier research also had to be withdrawn.

Primarily because of his remarkable output of papers, someone at the perpetrator's medical school had proposed him for a faculty appointment. After our findings came to light, however, he was dismissed. Since government funds were involved, we reported our conclusions to the U.S. attorney general's office. Ours was an investigation based on science, but we were aware that our findings had serious legal implications. In the background throughout our work were lawyers—for the accused, for the medical school, for the NIH itself. Our panel reviewed the circumstances of our inquiry with the president of the university in question. We recommended to the NIH that we return to the medical school following a year's probation to check that appropriate supervisory changes had been instituted. This we did, concluding that the school had dealt with the matter satisfactorily.

While we might debate the particular circumstances of each occurrence of falsification of research data and the motivation or psychological aberration of the individual concerned, such incidents emphasize the obligations of all concerned for the proper conduct of research. This includes the supervision of trainees, the retention of primary data, the regular scrutiny by experienced scientists of primary data and subsequent calculations, and the encouragement of free scientific interchange and exchange of data. Each author whose name appears on a manuscript must accept responsibility for its content. As a result of our investigation, some medical journals have established policies that all authors must provide at the time of a paper's submission written evidence that they accept such responsibility for the work.

Scientific misconduct may constitute fabrication, falsification, or plagiarism. In response to the NIH request, our panel of senior investigators recommended that when a serious wrongdoing is clear, the other scientific activities of the individual be investigated and key people and organizations be informed, including collaborators in continuing research projects; coauthors of papers, whether submitted for publication, in press, or already published; and those granting agencies with which the individual was involved at the time the data falsification occurred and those funding the individual's current research.

Each of these individuals and granting agencies must use moral and legal judgment in the way they respond to such information. If the complexity of the case indicates the issue cannot be resolved rapidly, the responsible institutional official must decide whether collaborators, coauthors, and granting agencies should be notified in confidence of the situation.

One consequence of cases such as these is the advent of whistle-blowers. A 1986 revision to the Civil War–era Federal False Claims Act, which punished military contractors and suppliers who defrauded the government, permits whistle-blowers to sue institutions suspected of fraud when research has been supported by federal funds. Because whistle-blowers may recover up to three times the amount of the federal funds involved, the law may actually encourage "bounty hunter" lawsuits aimed at institutions engaged in legitimate scientific research.

The long series of events involving David Baltimore is a case in point. Baltimore won the Nobel Prize in physiology or medicine in 1975 for his study of how a special class of viruses reproduces. A whistle-blower at the Massachusetts Institute of Technology, where he worked, accused one of Baltimore's coauthors on a 1986 paper in the journal *Cell* of falsifying data. The study, in which Baltimore had collaborated, was supported by NIH funds. The Office of Research Integrity within the office of the Assistant Secretary for Health upheld a preliminary finding of guilt and proposed to bar Baltimore's collaborator from receiving government funds for ten years, despite the usual penalty of three to five years.

The issue dragged on for a decade, a long, unhappy sequence of allegations, investigations, and appeals. A federal appeals panel finally ended the matter when it found that the Office of Research Integrity had failed to prove its charges "by a preponderance of the evidence." The panel recommended that no penalties be imposed on the accused. Nonetheless, the MIT whistle-blower received acclaim, including the Humanist of the Year award from the Ethical Society of Boston.

the Soviet Union

My continued interest in medical research on the heart and blood circulation has led me into many interesting experiences, not the least of which involved my participation with a U.S. scientific delegation to the Soviet Union during the 1980s. As a member of the Mayo Clinic staff well known for research in this area, I was asked to join the delegation. Our meetings alternated between sites in the United States and in the Soviet Union.

Our meetings in the United States were more or less uneventful, but for those in the Soviet Union the FBI interviewed us before we left the United

States and after our return. (The KGB always accompanied us wherever we went in the Soviet Union.) Our first meeting in the Soviet Union was with our colleagues at the USSR Cardiology Research Center in Moscow, followed by meetings in Leningrad (St. Petersburg), Kiev in the Ukraine, and Kaunas in Lithuania.

In the seventy-year history of the Soviet Union, spying was an ever-present fear, and visitors assumed they must be careful of what they said, since the KGB might well have bugged their hotel rooms. One story I heard concerned an American tourist who was convinced his Moscow hotel room was bugged. Pulling back the carpet, he found some bolts set into the floor. Believing he had located a bug, he removed the bolts and went to bed satisfied. "How did you sleep?" he asked the others in his group at breakfast the next morning. "I was OK—until the chandelier fell on my head!" answered a colleague.

I did not encounter spies so far as I am aware, but on one occasion I experienced a minor fainting spell as we had dinner with our Soviet colleagues in a Moscow restaurant. I lay on the floor for a short time as the Soviets suggested to the chair of our delegation that perhaps I go to a hospital. All of us in the U.S. delegation were concerned that Soviet hospitals might use unsterilized syringes containing viruses that cause severe liver damage. I soon recovered and said emphatically that I did not need to go to a hospital. The delegation chair took me back to our hotel, saw me into bed, and had a colleague stay with me. As I knew from the early work of my first teacher in research, Henry Barcroft, the drop in arterial blood pressure that causes a healthy subject to faint is due to the sudden dilatation of the arterial vessels in the skeletal muscles in the limbs. But what brought on my fainting spell? That remains a mystery, since it is still a challenge to determine just what precipitates a drop in arterial blood pressure.

The Russians are well known for the quantity of vodka they consume, and I can say that their reputation is well deserved. Early each morning, after breakfast but before the scientific meeting, our hosts served vodka. By tradition, you are to empty each glass in one gulp. One morning, after about an hour of this, I—intoxicated—happened to notice that one of my colleagues suffered no ill effects. When I asked him how he could remain sober, he showed me a rubber hot-water bottle that he wore under his shirt. With each "Bottoms up!" he simply disposed of the vodka by pouring it through an open shirt button into the bottle.

On another occasion, Vladislov Solovyev, a Soviet host whom we invited to the United States, wished to be polite and conform to American custom, as we had observed Russian customs in his country. We arranged a lunch meeting in New York with several prominent American citizens. Recalling the "Bottoms up!" that he had heard us speak before each gulp of vodka, Solovyev raised his glass to toast us and said, "Up your bottoms!"

I made lasting friends from my work with the Soviet delegation, including Vladimir Khayutin, a professor at the National Cardiology Research Center at the USSR Academy of Medical Sciences in Moscow, and his wife, Natalia Kaverina, chief of the academy's Laboratory of Cardiovascular Pharmacology. When their grandson, Nicolaus, was diagnosed with acute lymphocytic leukemia, I received an urgent message from Vladimir, asking if I could send leucovorin, an active form of the B-complex vitamin folate that's used in combination with chemotherapy because it promotes the normal formation of blood cells. With help from my Mayo colleagues in oncology, I dispatched a supply to my friends' Moscow apartment, but the shipment never arrived.

In desperation, I called an acquaintance at TWA, who assured me he would arrange delivery of the drug. Several days later, however, a TWA representative in Moscow called to say that the authorities said that the shipment could not be delivered since there was no one of that name at the address. I then gave the caller from TWA the address of the research center where my friends worked, and the package was sent there by private messenger. Thus, the supply of leucovorin finally reached Vladimir and Natalia. Sadly, little Nicolaus, their only grandchild, died a few years later, in 1987.

the Wolf Foundation

In 1978, about a decade after the Mideast hijacking episode involving Moni Samueloff, another Mayo alumnus, Henry N. Neufeld, invited me to help select the winners of the 1979 Wolf Prize in medicine. Neufeld was then director of the Heart Institute at Tel-Hasomer Hospital in Tel Aviv.

The Wolf Foundation was created in 1978 by Ricardo Subirana Lobo Wolf, a German-born inventor who had made a fortune in business in South America before settling in Cuba before World War I, created the Wolf Foundation in 1978. Wolf became a diplomat in an unusual fashion. A wealthy man living in Cuba, Wolf needed Fidel Castro's permission to retire to Israel. Castro not only gave his permission but also appointed him in 1961—after Wolf said he would build a suitable residence at his own expense—as Cuba's ambassador to Israel. How much Israel needed a Cuban embassy we don't know, but Wolf and his wife, Francisca, moved to Israel and built a beautiful home in Hertzlia on the shores of the Mediterranean, north of Tel Aviv. Wolf added the English translation of his surname, Lobo, to his name after he came to Israel.

Every year, the Wolf Foundation awards five or six $100,000 prizes on an international basis in agriculture, arts, chemistry, mathematics, medicine, and physics. Wolf provided that the prize winners would be selected by committees "comprising world-renowned scientists and experts in each field." Whenever possible, the selection committee is to include a Nobel laureate. The 1979 committee on which I served included Baruch S. Blumberg of the Institute for Cancer Research in Philadelphia, who shared the 1976 Nobel Prize in physiology or medicine with Irving Millman for their work with infectious diseases.

We selected three recipients: Roger W. Sperry of the California Institute of Technology in Pasadena for his studies on the functional differentiation of the right and left hemispheres of the brain; Arvid Carlsson of the University of Göteborg in Sweden for his work establishing the role of dopamine as a neurotransmitter; and Oleh Hornykiewicz of the University of Vienna in Austria for opening a new approach in the control of Parkinson's disease with L-dopa.

The Wolf Prizes are presented in an impressive ceremony at the Chagall Hall of the Knesset Building and attended by the president of Israel, the speaker of the Knesset, and usually the prime minister. Following the 1979 ceremony, all proceeded to the Wolf home for a reception.

When the Knesset first approved the Wolf Foundation, the members of the Israeli Academy of Sciences hoped the awards would be limited to Israeli citizens. No Israelis had been selected by the time I participated in the process. Asked to chair the committee for the following year, I invited Konrad Bloch of Harvard University and Nathan Treinin of the Weizmann Institute of Science in Israel to join me. We again selected three recipients: Ceser Milstein (later a Nobel laureate) and his colleague Sir James Gowan of the Medical Research Council in Cambridge and London, as well as Leo Sachs of the Weizmann Institute of Science, for their contributions about cells through their studies on the immunological role of the lymphocytes, the development of specific antibodies, and the mechanisms that govern the control and differentiation of normal and cancer cells. The winners shared the $100,000 award equally. I especially enjoyed seeing Sachs, a distinguished (and deserving) Israeli, receive the award.

I am grateful to the Mayo Clinic for supporting my participation in important national and international events, such as with the U.S. space program, and for granting leave with pay during those times I was away from my Mayo responsibilities. Such an arrangement not only brings recognition and credit to the clinic, but also follows the examples of paid leaves set by Mayo's founders. And yet, as rewarding as my extramural commitments were during the late 1960s and early 1970s, I was genuinely excited in 1977 to turn my full attention to my new responsibilities as Mayo's director for education and dean of its new medical school.

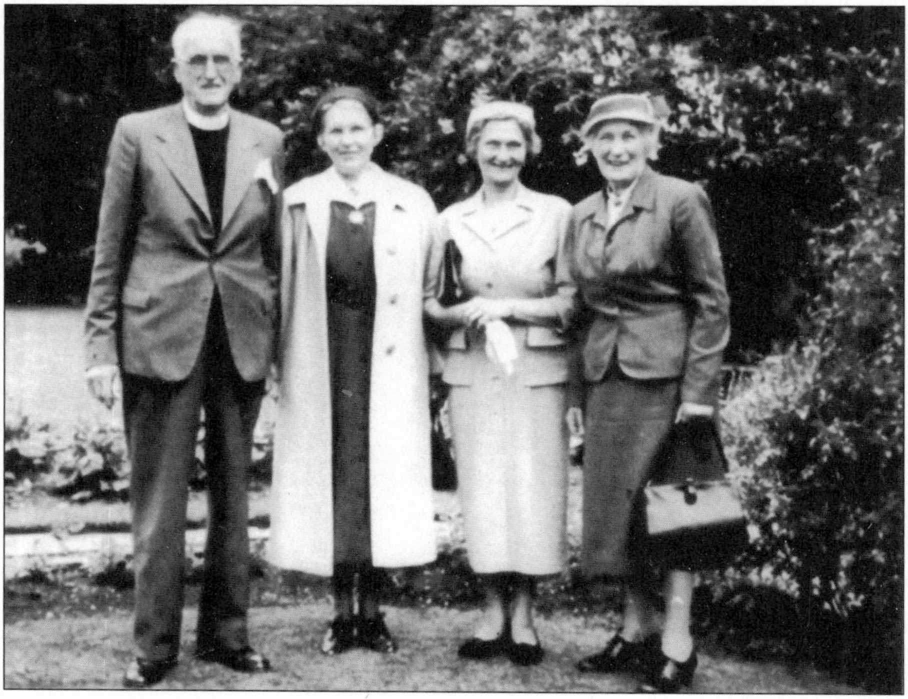

From left: My father, the Reverend William Frederick Shepherd; my Aunt Lena; my mother, Matilda (Tilly) Shepherd; and my mother-in-law, Jane Johnston.

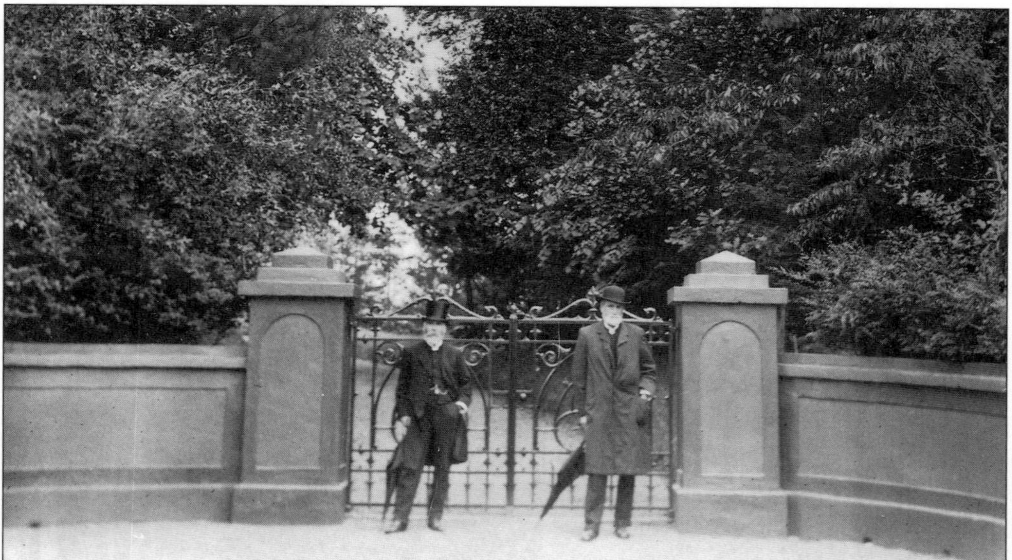

Relative Robert Kirk (left) and my grandfather, William Shepherd, stand at the entry to Kirk's Belfast mansion, "The Pines."

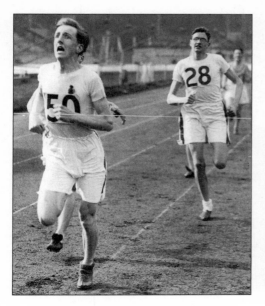

I won the half-mile race in the semifinals of the Public Schools Athletic Competition but lost the finals the next day (wearing jersey number 28).

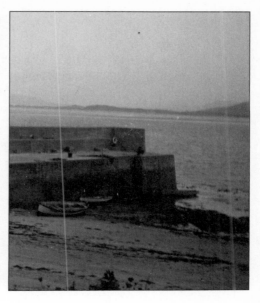

The pier in Portnoo in County Donegal from which I dove into the sea to impress Helen Mary Johnston, my future wife.

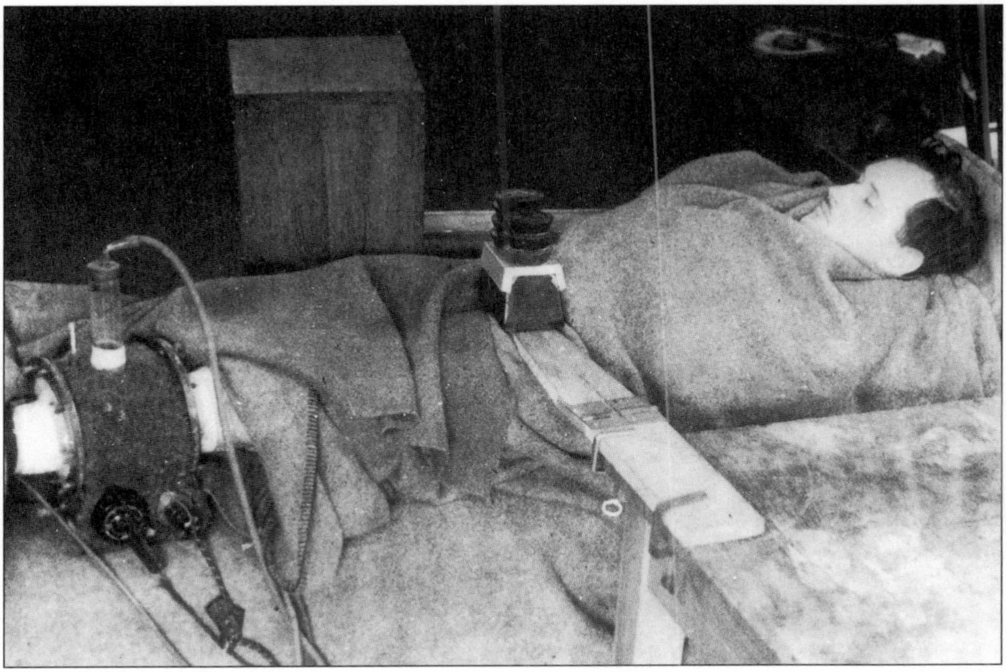

During my years as a researcher I was often a subject in medical experiments, including this one to measure blood flow to the left leg.

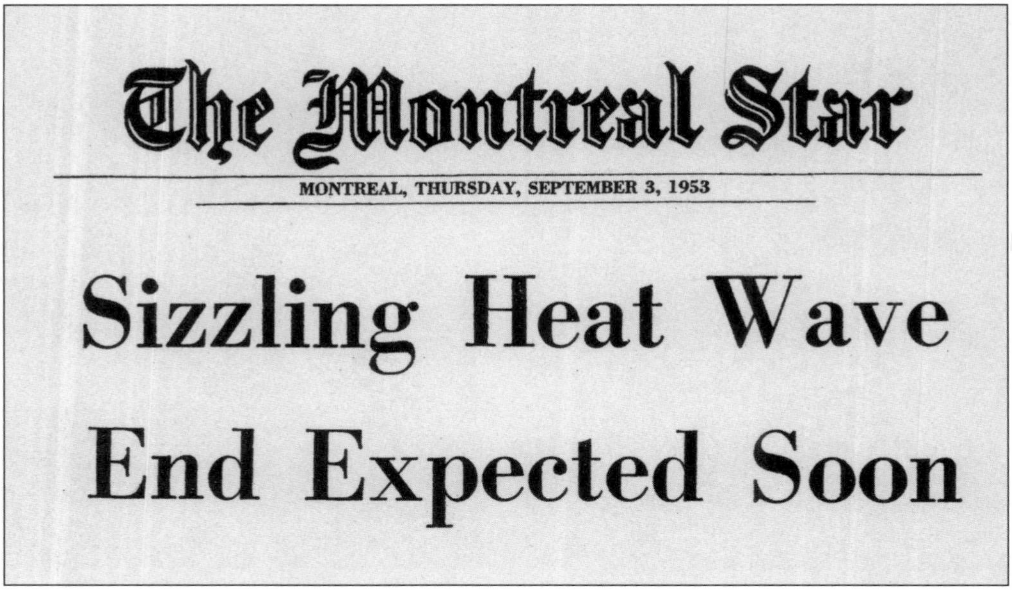

The Montreal Star

MONTREAL, THURSDAY, SEPTEMBER 3, 1953

Sizzling Heat Wave End Expected Soon

A record heat wave swept over Montreal as the Shepherd family arrived in North America for the first time in September 1953.

After my year's sabbatical at the Mayo Clinic, Gillian, Roger, Helen and I sailed back to England in 1954 aboard the *Queen Mary*.

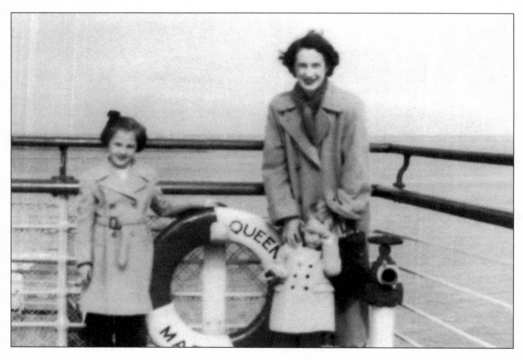

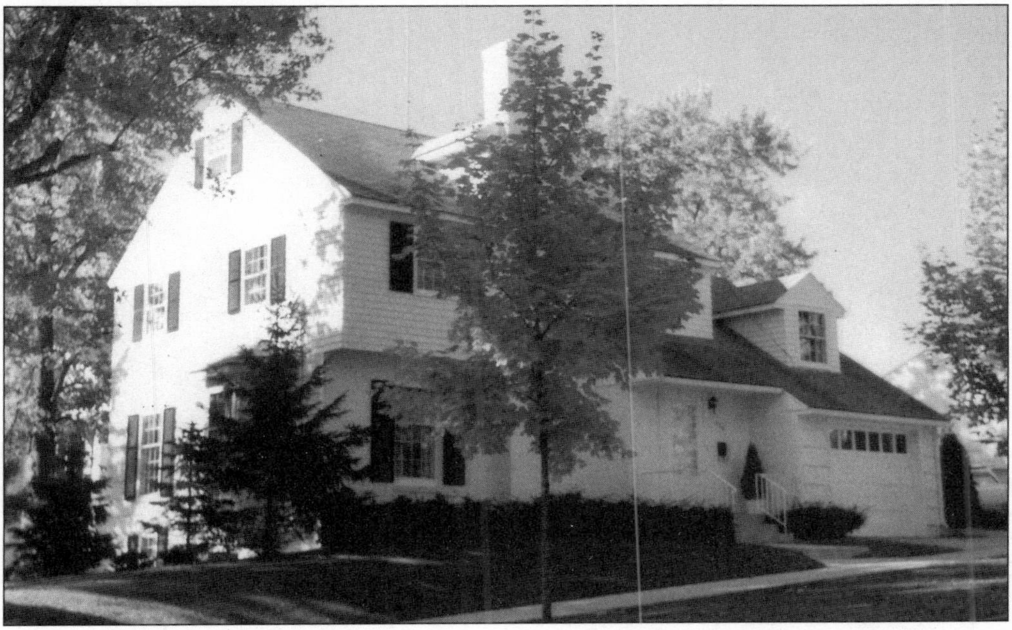

The Shepherd home in southwest Rochester, Minnesota, an area known locally as "Pill Hill."

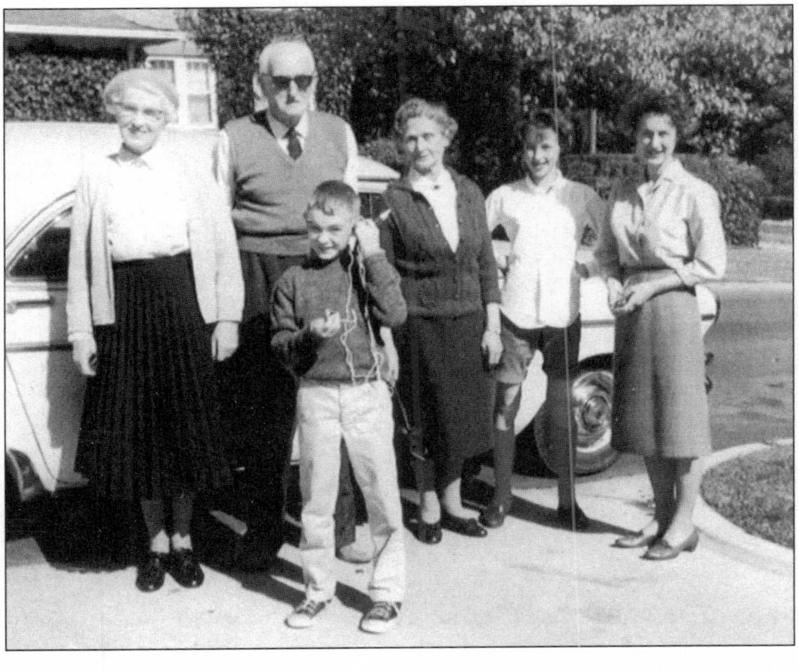

My family visited from Ireland after we settled in Rochester. From left: Aunt Lena; father William; mother Tilly; and Gillian, Helen, and Roger (foreground).

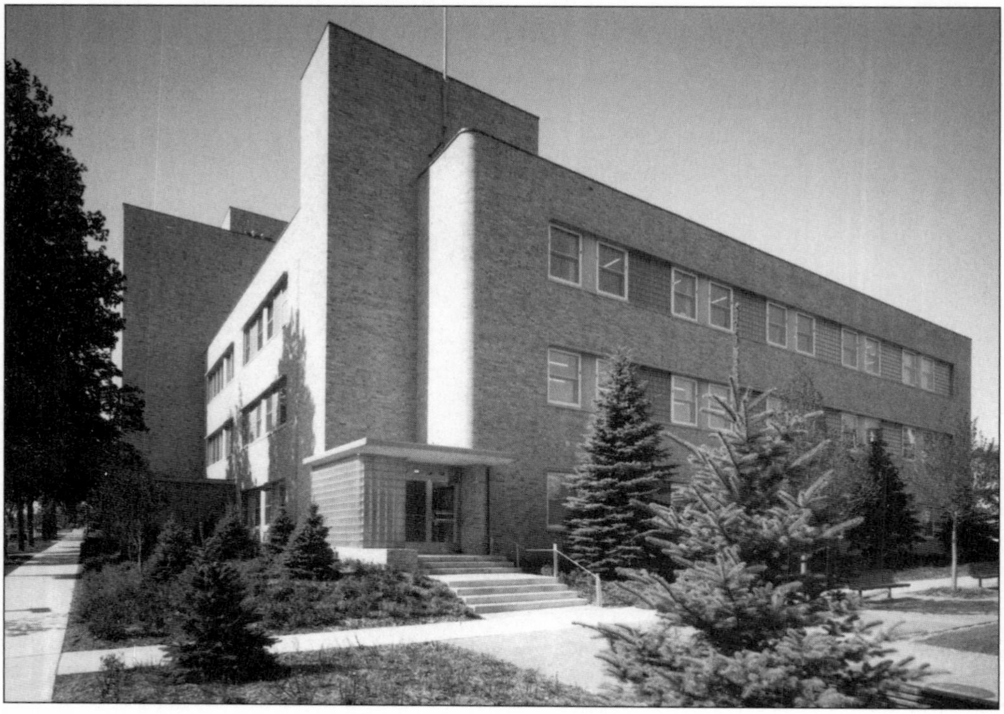

The expanded Medical Sciences Building at the Mayo Clinic in Rochester. (MAYO PHOTO ARCHIVES)

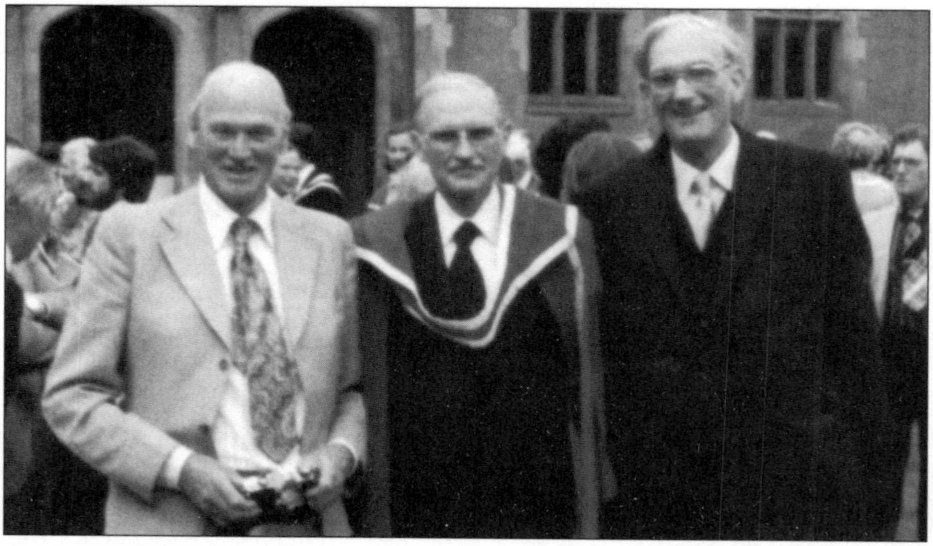

My older brothers and I reunite at Queen's University in Belfast in July 1979 after I receive an honorary doctorate of science. From left: Harry ("Shepherd Major"), John ("Shepherd Minimus"), and Fred ("Shepherd Minor").

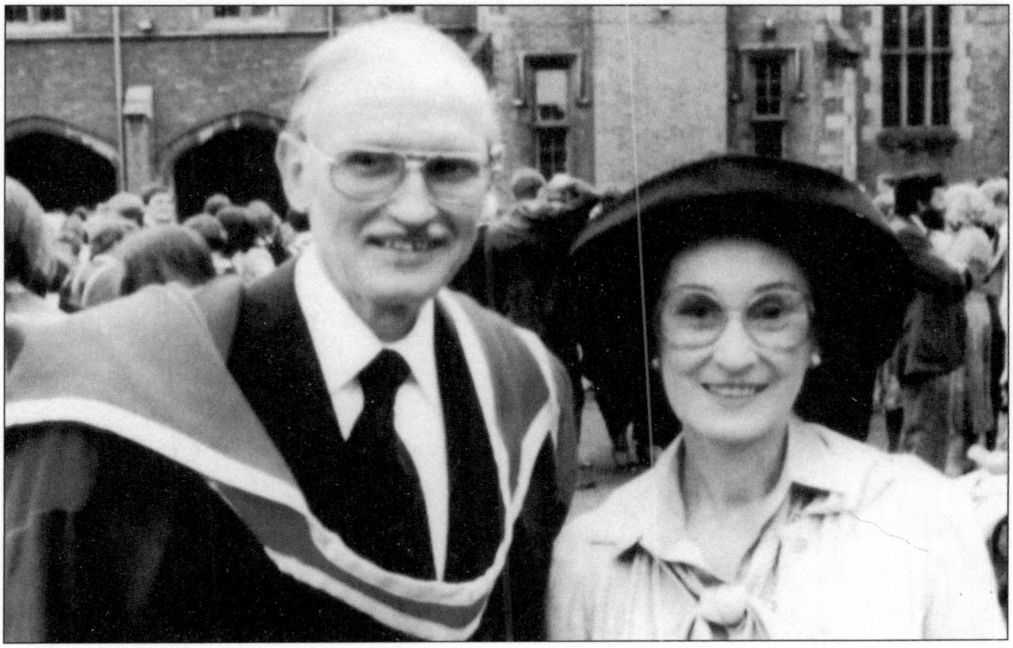

Helen accompanied me to Queen's University when I accepted my honorary doctorate of science.

JOHN T. SHEPHERD, M.D., M.Ch., D.Sc.
Professor of Physiology, Mayo Medical School and Mayo Graduate School of Medicine (University of Minnesota), Director for Research, Mayo Foundation, Rochester, Minnesota, USA.

PAUL M. VANHOUTTE, M.D., Ag.E.S.
Professor of Physiology, Department of Internal Medicine, Universitaire Instelling Antwerpen, Wilrijk, Belgium. Formerly, Research Associate, Department of Physiology and Biophysics, Mayo Clinic and Mayo Foundation, Rochester, Minnesota, USA.

Veins and their Control

1975
W. B. Saunders Company Ltd London · Philadelphia · Toronto

I collaborated with research fellow Paul Vanhoutte on the 1975 book *Veins and Their Control.*

The Human Cardiovascular System

Facts and Concepts

John T. Shepherd, M.D., M.Ch., D.Sc., F.R.C.P.
Professor of Physiology and Dean
Mayo Medical School
and Director for Education
Mayo Foundation
Rochester, Minnesota

Paul M. Vanhoutte, M.D., Ag.E.S.
Professor of Pharmacology and Pathophysiology
Department of Medicine
Universitaire Instelling Antwerpen
University of Antwerp
Wilrijk, Belgium

Raven Press • New York 1979

Dedication

To Dr. L. Vandendriessche, formerly Rector of the Universitaire Instelling Antwerpen, and the Board of Trustees of the Francqui Foundation, Brussels: the former for sponsoring Dr. Shepherd for an International Francqui Chair at the University of Antwerp and the latter for providing the award. These events permitted two long-time colleagues to continue their collaboration in research and to develop the groundwork for this overview of the cardiovascular system.

I again collaborated with Paul Vanhoutte on *The Human Cardiovascular System* in 1979.

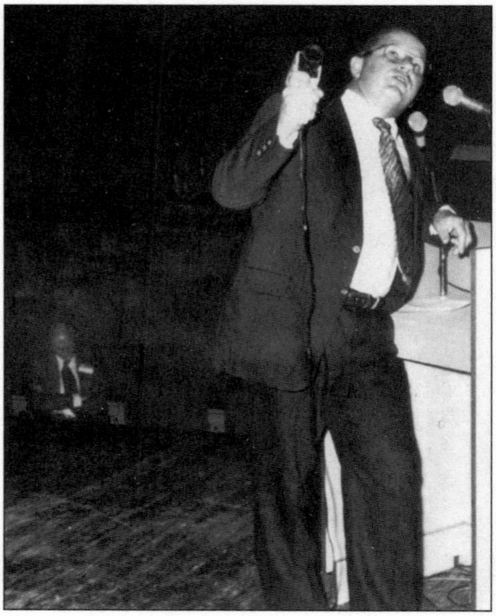

Paul Vanhoutte gives a lecture in 1979 in Paris. Note that I, the second invited speaker, appear to be asleep in the front row (to Paul's left).

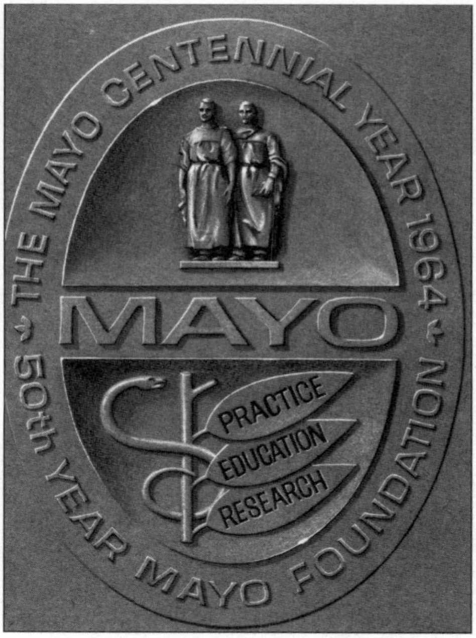

The Mayo Foundation marked its fiftieth anniversary in 1969. (MAYO PHOTO ARCHIVES)

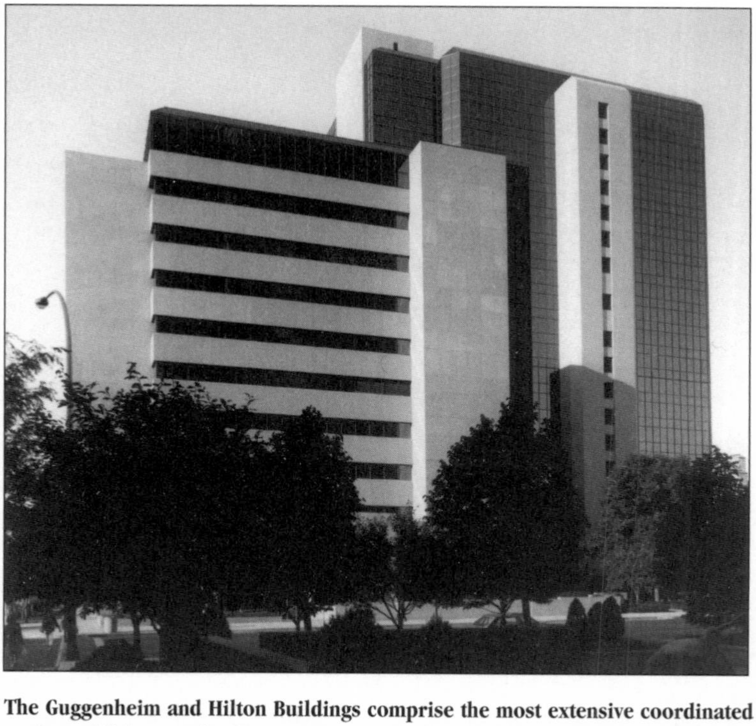

The Guggenheim and Hilton Buildings comprise the most extensive coordinated project additions to the Mayo campus in Rochester. (MAYO PHOTO ARCHIVES)

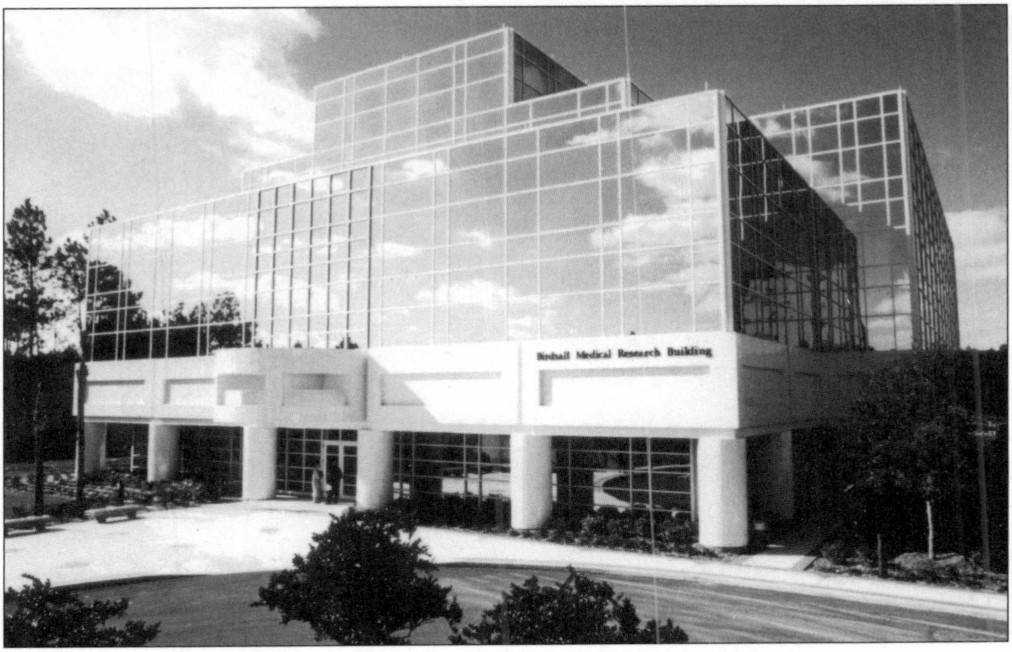

The Birdsall Medical Research Building at Mayo Clinic Jacksonville. (MAYO PHOTO ARCHIVES)

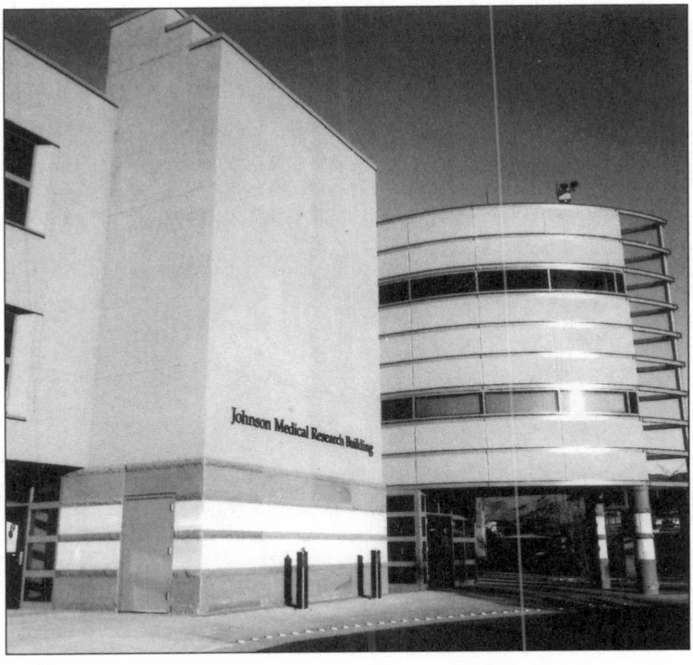

The Johnson Medical Research Building at Mayo Clinic Scottsdale. (MAYO PHOTO ARCHIVES)

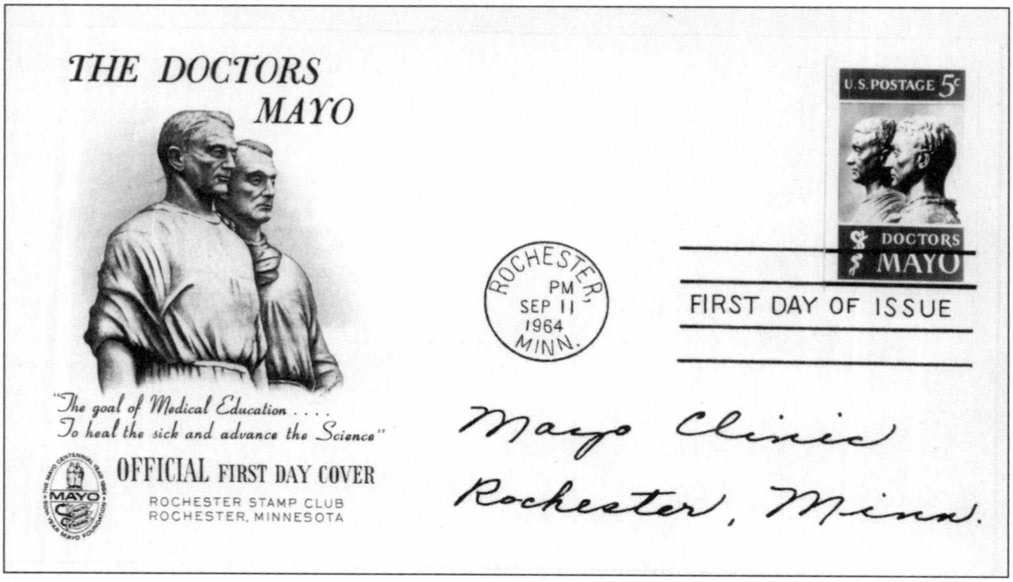

At the suggestion of photographer Clarence Stearns of Rochester, the postal service issued a stamp on September 11, 1964, honoring William J. and Charles H. Mayo upon the centennial of the clinic.

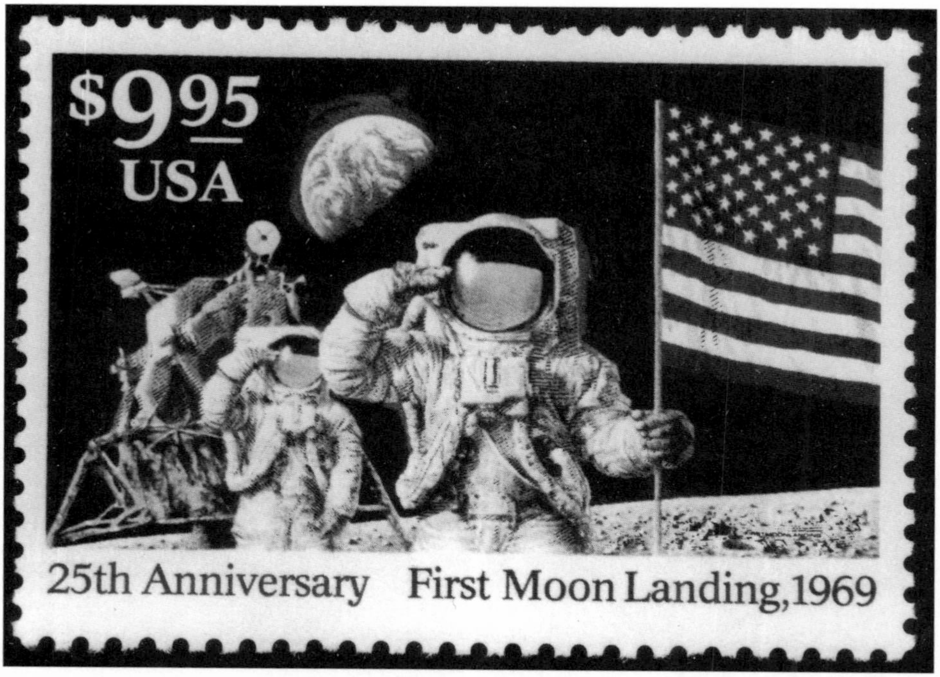

The U.S. Postal Service commemorated America's moon landing in July 1969 with a stamp to cover express postage. It features astronauts Neil Armstrong and Buzz Aldrin Jr.

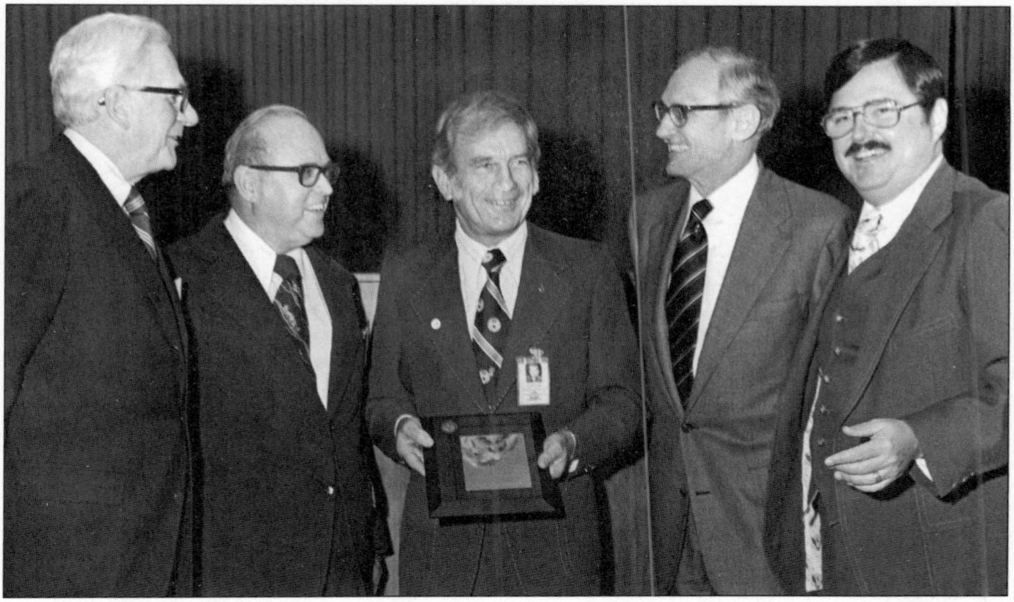

As American Heart Association president I presented astronaut Deke Slayton (center) the "Heart of the Year" Award in October 1976 at the Johnson Space Center in Houston. He piloted the *Apollo-Soyuz,* a joint American-Soviet space flight mission, in July 1975. From left: AHA executive vice president William Moore, Texas AHA president Edwin Morrow, Slayton, John Shepherd, and Texas AHA public relations committee chair Frank Weaver.

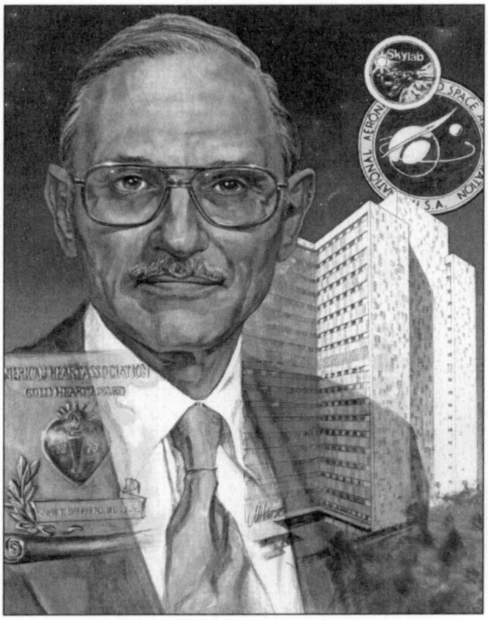

I received NASA's Skylab Achievement Award in 1974.

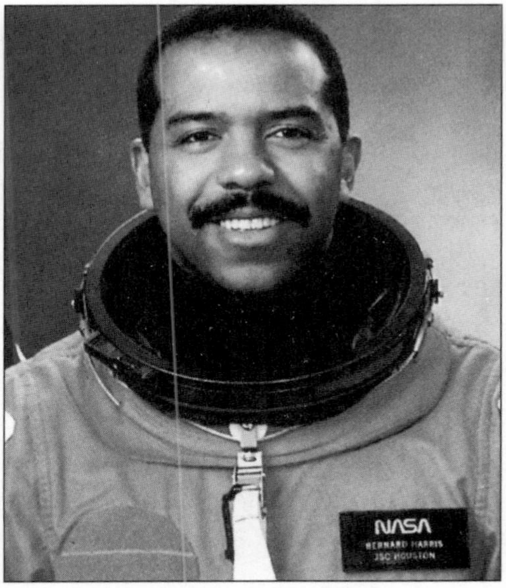

During an eight-day flight of the shuttle *Discovery* in 1995, Bernard Harris, a 1985 graduate of Mayo's internal medicine residency program, was the first African American to walk in space.

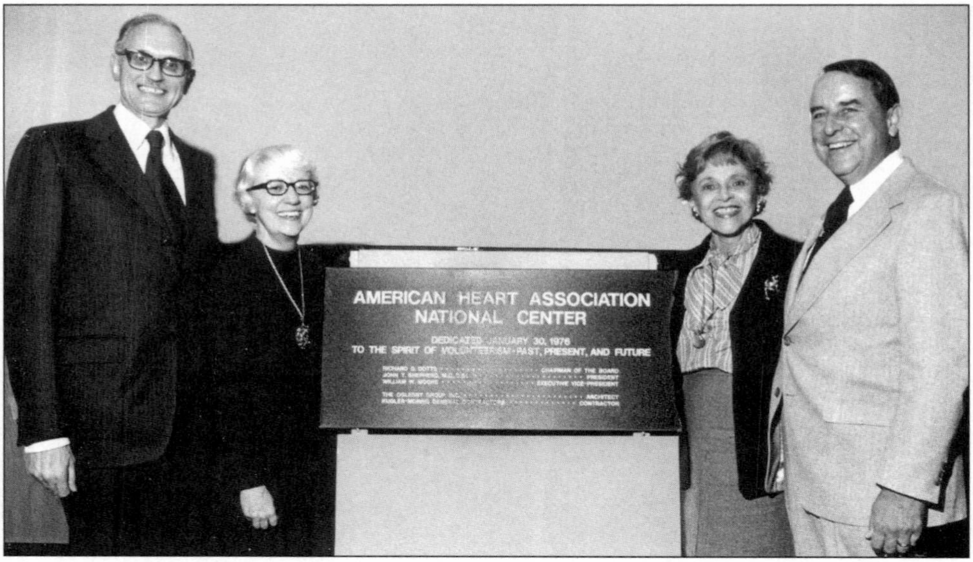

As president of the American Heart Association, I dedicated the AHA National Center in Dallas in 1976. With me, from left: Harriet Dustan, who succeeded me as AHA president; Mrs. Andrew Fraser, a representative of the Texas AHA affiliate; and Richard Dotts, past AHA board chair.

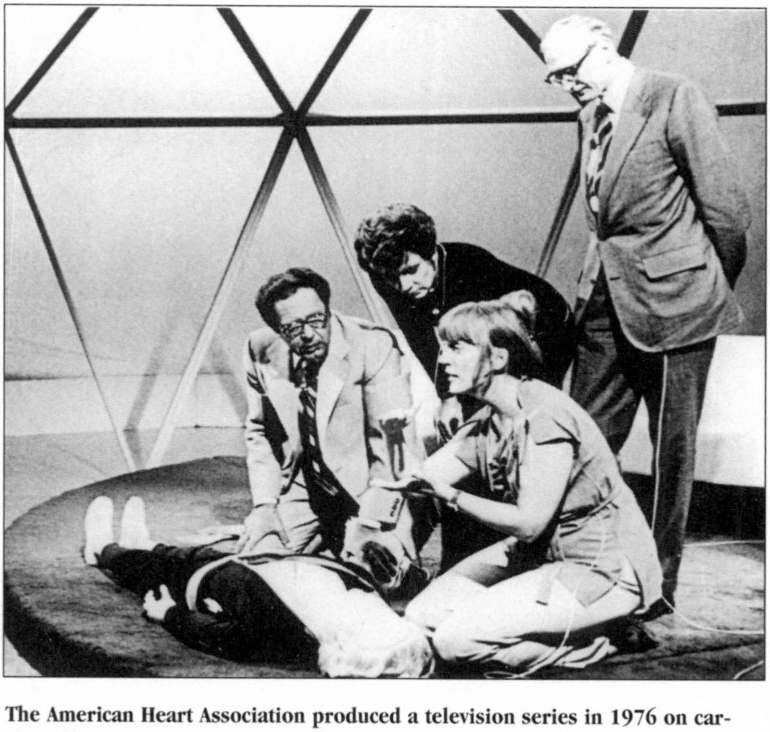

The American Heart Association produced a television series in 1976 on cardiopulmonary resuscitation. As AHA president, I (standing) observed a demonstration of the procedure.

4

launching Mayo's medical school

My six years as director for education at Mayo coincided with groundbreaking events in the clinic's history. Between 1977 and 1983, my administrative colleagues and I faced significant challenges, not the least of which was establishing Mayo's fully accredited medical school, of which I later became dean. In the process of opening the school, we also closed a significant chapter in Mayo's history: a sixty-six-year affiliation with the University of Minnesota medical school.

As my role as director for education evolved, I kept in mind the words of several sages on the topic. One was former president Lyndon Johnson, a member of Mayo's board of trustees from 1969 to 1973. Johnson once said he had learned one great truth in life – that the answer to all the world's problems came down to a single word: education.

On the subject of medical education specifically, nineteenth-century Irish physician William Stokes offered these words: "Let us emancipate the student and give him time and opportunity for the cultivation of his mind, so that in his pupilage he not be a puppet in the hands of others, but rather a self-relying and reflecting being." Charles H. Mayo was especially prophetic when he said, "Today the only thing that is permanent is change. The people will gradually demand more of their medical advisors. Probably in the not-too-distant future, we will crawl out of our old methods of education (as a snake sheds its skin) and reorganize a new plan."

The new plan that led to opening Mayo's medical school was firmly envisioned within the context of the clinic's past endeavors in education – endeavors that demonstrated the remarkable foresight of Drs. Charles and Will Mayo.

Mayo's history in education

Mayo Clinic carries on the principle established by its founders that continuing medical education should be a priority. It's a tradition that began when the Mayo brothers first proposed an affiliation between their clinic and the University of Minnesota in 1913. After arranging an agreement on June 9, 1915, the Mayo brothers gave the University of Minnesota $1.5 million for the Mayo Foundation for Medical Education and Research. According to Dr. Will Mayo, the agreement stipulated that the sum should reach $2 million or more before any part of the money were used.

Academic affiliation with the University of Minnesota provided the bulwark for the development of academic programs at Mayo. According to pathologist Louis B. Wilson, first director of the Mayo Foundation, the development of educational standards for graduate degrees in medical specialties "has proceeded so satisfactorily since the Mayo Foundation became part of the Graduate School of the University of Minnesota that these standards have received national recognition by all medical specialty boards, all of which have been formed during the last quarter century."

Some private practitioners opposed the affiliation of the clinic with the university, however, viewing the group practice at Mayo as a threat to their incomes. Opponents took their objections to the Minnesota legislature, where a bill was introduced instructing the university's board of regents to dissolve the affiliation between the graduate school and the Mayo Foundation. Finally, on March 22, 1917, Will Mayo appeared before the Senate Committee on Education, which was conducting public hearings on the bill. As reported in the *Minneapolis Morning Tribune* on March 24, he told why he and his brother had offered their gift of service and money to the state.

"We never take [debt] notes. No mortgage has ever been given on a home to pay a bill here. We never sue. Thirty percent of our patients are charity cases," began Dr. Will, who paid tribute to his father, William Worrall Mayo, for inspiring the ideals that had guided the brothers. "My father kept a common pocketbook with his boys, each using it as his wishes required. After my father died, my brother and I continued the common pocketbook. We realized that all we are and all we have we owe to the people of Minnesota, and we consider that we are holding this fund in trust for the 2,500,000 people of this state, and we want to return it to them." His extemporaneous remarks were so powerful and eloquent that support for the bill subsided rapidly. The affiliation between Mayo and the University of Minnesota became permanent on September 13, 1917.

There could be no doubt that the Mayo brothers "recognized certain definite social obligations" inherited from their father, as Will Mayo later wrote to university president L. D. Coffman on February 15, 1934. W. W. Mayo believed that any man who had greater opportunity, or who had greater physical, intellectual, or moral strength, owed something to those less fortunate; that is, he believed that each of us needs to carry his or her own share of responsibility. Dr. Will acknowledged the unique opportunity he and Charles had received. Each traveled at home and abroad to study subjects connected with surgery, as well as to attend medical meetings, while the other could stay at home carrying on the practice.

Although new staff members at Mayo received a salary, there was no profit sharing. Beginning in 1894, the brothers set aside money from their earnings to do "something worthwhile for the sick," which they invested until the fund had grown far beyond their expectations. (Although endowment of the Mayo Foundation had increased to more than $5 million by the time I became Mayo director for education in 1977, the interest generated no longer met the stipend requirements of the fellows.) Since the money had come from the sick, Will Mayo wrote Coffman, he and his brother believed it ought to return to the sick through advanced medical education, which would develop better physicians, and to research, which would reduce the amount of disease.

Will concluded his letter to President Coffman by announcing that Mayo would add $500,000 to the endowment of the Mayo Foundation at the university, claiming that he and Charlie had merely been moral custodians of the people's money. Of the letter, Coffman wrote: "Seldom in anyone's lifetime does the opportunity come to read a document as sincere, mature in philosophy, and yet unpretentious. . . . Composed by a man who has been honored in every part of the world, it reveals the heart and thought of one at the peak of his profession who has never lost touch with the simple verities of life, or in achieving success failed to appreciate his obligations to his profession and the society in which he has practiced it."

degrees in the medical sciences

At the time of Mayo's letter to Coffman, no funds were available for those wishing advanced training in medicine in the United States. Mayo Graduate School, therefore, represented an attractive possibility for outstanding candidates from around the world. The school benefited Mayo as well, for top graduates often were invited to join the staff. In addition, the clinic's affiliation with the university permitted trainees to take a master's or doctoral degree, each of which demanded a thesis based on original studies. These degree programs encourage each trainee to learn more of the science of medicine. (No small feat, when you consider that an estimated two million articles appear in twenty thousand scientific journals worldwide each year!) In fact, after the graduate program began, those invited to join the Mayo clinical staff customarily had earned the master of science degree and those joining the medical sciences, a doctorate.

During the 1930s and 1940s, University of Minnesota chair of surgery Owen Wangensteen and chair of physiology Maurice Visscher had established an outstanding program for training future heart surgeons. They insisted that each trainee achieve a doctorate in the medical sciences to ensure originality in future work. Successful candidates became leaders in cardiac surgery in the United States and elsewhere. One, Christiaan Barnard, returned to Cape Town, South Africa, where he performed the world's first human heart transplant on December 3, 1967.

postwar housing for graduates

After the end of World War II, thousands of young physicians sought additional training in the United States, many of them at the Mayo Clinic. Along with them came staff physicians returning after discharge from military service and many Mayo research fellows whose training had been interrupted by the war. Housing in Rochester, as elsewhere in United States in the late 1940s, was in critically short supply.

In response, Mayo built three housing additions: Homestead Addition in southeast Rochester, Carroll Addition in northeast Rochester, and prefabricated units in southwest Rochester. Staff physicians and fellows could purchase homes in Homestead and Carroll, but the prefabs were Quonset huts reserved for rent by Mayo fellows with families that included at least one child.

The quickly constructed prefabs consisted of one-story living quarters above concrete basements. Despite their crude, temporary nature—the units were built to last about ten years—residents who lived in them quickly developed into a close-knit community. Such was the prefabs' popularity, in fact, that until 1950 the waiting list sometimes ran to more than one hundred applicants. Even after the pressure for housing declined in the early 1950s, some fellows sought their friendly atmosphere. One alumnus recalled that the prefabs, which he called "chicken coops," were a place where "everybody was in the same boat—on the G.I. Bill, all semi-broke, with children, all of us trying to learn everything there was to know."

The Quonsets were identical in shape and size, about the only difference being the color of the roof tile. Not surprisingly, the many children living in the huts (the community soon became known as "Fertility Valley") sometimes ran into the wrong house on urgent bathroom missions. Confused by the similarity of the buildings, they might encounter a stranger there for the same purpose!

When the dam of the Zumbro River at Mayowood, the former home of Charles Mayo, burst after a torrential rain in July 1951, a wall of water descended into the low-lying area of the prefab homes. Many basements flooded and eventually some walls caved in. By the early 1960s, the Quonsets had exceeded their life span. With asphalt tile roofs and poor insulation, they were too hot in the summer and too cold in the winter. Many were sold to area farmers, who used them for living accommodations or storage sheds. Mayo residents gradually moved into more permanent structures.

During the late 1960s and early 1970s, many Mayo residents felt increasingly unhappy as they spent long hours carrying out clinical responsibilities and had too little time for academic study. In addition, their stipends did not match those of residents at other institutions. Dissatisfaction reached a head in the spring of 1971. At the time, I was director for research, Raymond Pruitt was director for education, and Emmerson Ward was chair of the board of governors. The residents chose a colleague as their spokesperson. He made frequent visits to each of us, urging changes. We agreed that changes were appropriate, and Pruitt wrote a letter on May 4, 1971, to that effect to the Mayo staff and fellows regarding stipends and other related matters.

A subcommittee of the Residency Review Committee took up the question and put it on the board of trustees' agenda. "Good progress was being made in establishing a proposed new stipend schedule, for residency training, and for research assistants and research associates," according to the staff newsletter of May 14. "It had been hoped that this new schedule would be implemented July 1, 1971."

Before we could take action, however, we received a letter from a Minneapolis law firm retained by the Association of Fellows, requesting a meeting to negotiate stipends, insurance, duties for fellows, on-call schedules, meals, vacation, parking privileges, and more. Ward, Pruitt, and I advised the fellows that the appearance of an attorney made it inappropriate to continue discussions of these matters. All ended well after the fellows withdrew their legal representative.

Mayo Medical School

The idea that Mayo might be the center of a new medical school in Minnesota followed a decade-long examination of medical education in the state. Beginning in the late 1960s, people throughout the country began to see the need for more doctors. The University of Minnesota Medical School responded by rapidly increasing its enrollment, and the university's board of regents began to investigate the possibility of expanding medical education in the state, including a larger teaching role at Mayo. Gradually, "members of the profession and lay citizens alike began thinking of the possibilities for a new medical school or schools," according to Slade Schuster, chair of the Mayo Department of Administration and a member of the boards of governors and trustees. Writing in *Mayo Alumnus* in 1976, Schuster noted a frequently expressed public opinion: "If a second medical school is warranted in Minnesota, why not most logically and readily in Rochester?"

The Mayo Foundation asked John A. D. Cooper, dean of sciences at Northwestern University, to form a review panel to examine Mayo's educational programs. At the same time, Mayo and the University of Minnesota formed a commission of university presidents—chaired by Laurence M. Gould, president emeritus of Carleton College in Northfield, Minnesota—to look at establishing a medical school in Rochester. The Minnesota legislature meanwhile established an interim commission to study the questions of additional medical education in Minnesota, its location, and prospective dependence upon state funding.

The three groups made nearly unanimous recommendations: Mayo Foundation should establish, sponsor, and conduct a second medical school in association with the University of Minnesota. It should model the long-standing affiliation of the Mayo Graduate School of Medicine and the university. The affiliation should extend to include the new Mayo Medical School. (In addition, the legislative commission recommended consideration of a *third* school, at the University of Minnesota–Duluth, which was established in 1972.) As both Cooper's review panel and Gould's commission of university presidents noted, expanding into undergraduate medical education was essential for Mayo to round out its existing programs in medical research, graduate medical education, and health-sciences teaching.

The usual routine of Mayo's board of governors regarding complex issues was to select committees to review different aspects of the question at hand. As a member of the board since 1966, I helped to name six such committees. The committee that looked at the advantages and disadvantages of a medical school concluded that it could approach a unanimous decision—*if* we could ensure outside financial support with control; federation with the University of Minnesota without loss of financial or administrative autonomy; considerable increase in the staff from outside the institution without creation of an academic hierarchy; continuation of our ideals of providing superior medical care to patients as our primary goal; and proper balance between undergraduate and postgraduate education. Another committee considered the potential financial impact on Mayo. A third, which I chaired, looked at potential curriculum. Other committees deliberated on the facilities required, the reaction of Mayo staff to teaching medical students, and the reaction of Mayo patients to the presence of medical students.

Some worried that the casual dress of medical students might upset Mayo patients. This concern arose from a long-established practice at Mayo that, except in the hospitals, clinical staff and residents not wear white coats when seeing patients in diagnostic buildings. The idea behind "white-coat hypertension" was that patients felt more comfortable when their physicians dressed more like them.

As Mayo discussed the merits of a medical school, the term "U.S. medical schools" as used by Congress became important. We watched carefully for the term, always requesting the additional words "including graduate schools of medicine." This may seem trivial, but we worried that Mayo could be deprived of financial or other benefit were the phrase not included.

The discussion proceeded, and the six committees presented a model of the nature, size, and curriculum of the proposed school at a meeting of the Mayo Foundation board of trustees in July 1968. Composed of both external members and members of the Mayo board of governors, the Mayo board of trustees is the ultimate decision-making body for the Mayo Clinic and Foundation. Based on costs and norms at other medical schools, we set the minimum number of students to justify a four-year school at forty per year. We calculated that the cost of educating each student would be $16,000 per year. When we brought the question of funding to the board of trustees, Warren Burger advised that we not take funds from our research or graduate education programs to support a medical school. Burger, an external trustee from 1959 until President Richard Nixon appointed him chief justice of the Supreme Court in 1969, proposed we raise enough funds from non-Mayo sources to support the school for its first ten years—about $33 million.

Based on his recommendation, the board of trustees made a hallmark decision: Mayo would attempt to raise all needed funds in the private sector. This was something totally new. The Mayos had found raising private funds neither necessary nor desirable. Still, we recalled something that Will Mayo once wrote: "It is necessary that each generation shall control its own destiny." To accomplish the ambitious fund-raising goal, Mayo established a board of development (which I joined in 1972 and became chair of in 1983) and soon raised the funds necessary to operate an undergraduate medical school for ten years.

At a news conference on November 12, 1971, Atherton Bean, chair of the Mayo board of trustees, announced that the board had unanimously approved the opening of Mayo Medical School. Raymond Pruitt, who had worked so hard to bring the new medical school into being, was its first dean. In the words of Malcolm Moos, then president of the University of Minnesota, it was "a tall moment." In its issue of July 4, 1976, the *Mayo Alumnus* identified three turning points for the future of the Mayo Clinic and Mayo Foundation: acceptance of external financing beginning in 1957, merger of the Mayo Clinic and Foundation in 1969, and establishment of the Mayo Medical School in 1972.

Before Mayo admitted the first class, it had to resolve a key question: Would the University of Minnesota provide academic support? This was important because we had proposed that the medical school operate under the auspices of the university and that the university would award medical degrees. When we asked university officials this question, they said their approval would be subject to a condition: the university must approve Mayo grant applications to the National Institutes of Health so as to avoid conflict with university applications. Such a condition would permit the university to veto any and all Mayo applications. We proposed instead that the NIH receive and review *all* applications and decide which merited funding. Only after Stephen Keating, chair of the Mayo board of trustees, met with his counterpart from the university was the matter settled. The university would omit the requirement and award the medical degree to graduates of Mayo Medical School. Mayo was free to make grant applications to the NIH without consulting the university.

Mayo sought funding for the medical school from the Minnesota legislature—a fixed amount of $8,000 per student—but no capital funding for building. Mayo needed support not just for the two years of a given biennium but for as long as it fulfilled its obligations under the appropriation. Surely that $8,000 per student was a bargain: the state would benefit from forty students entering the study of medicine each year.

Still, two elements in Mayo's proposal concerned legislators. First, although they acknowledged Mayo as a national resource in the field of health care and medical education, they did not believe it the responsibility of the people of Minnesota to provide support for nonstate residents. They limited the capitation act to Minnesota residents. Their second concern was more difficult. While they recognized Mayo as a tertiary care center with educational programs that had produced medical and surgical specialists for half a century, they wanted to expand the number of physicians providing primary care in the state's rural communities. Was Mayo concerned about producing specialists in family practice?

At one point, several legislators put forth a proposal for the capitation only of those Mayo students agreeing to enter family practice. In the end, however, Mayo affirmed that its medical educational programs would produce primary-care physicians as well as specialists. With the support of the chair of Mayo's Department of Internal Medicine and the dean of Mayo Medical School, the newly formed Mayo Medical Service Study Committee agreed that the school would include a Department of Family Medicine. Led by John R. Hodgson, chair of the Department of Radiology and a member of the Clinical Practice Committee, the Medical Service Study Committee also agreed that the Department of Family Medicine would work with the Minnesota Academy of Family Practice to develop educational resources for acquainting medical students with the responsibilities of family practice specialists.

After succeeding the first dean of the medical school, I appeared at intervals before the legislative committee overseeing annual capitation awards to justify continuing the state financial support. But no matter how prepared I might have been for this experience, I never could predict what questions legislators might ask.

first dean of Mayo Medical School

Mayo knew when it launched the medical school in September 1972 that its first dean, like the red heifer of the Israelites, must be free of blemish in the eyes of University of Minnesota colleagues and accrediting bodies. Raymond Pruitt filled the bill. A former Rhodes Scholar at Oxford University, Pruitt had been a Mayo resident in medicine and a staff cardiologist, then associate director of the Mayo Graduate School, professor and chair of the Department of Medicine at Baylor University's College of Medicine in Texas, and vice president of medical affairs at Baylor.

Pruitt, brought up in Arkansas, was happy to return to Mayo as the first dean of the medical school. He devised the curriculum and appointed the admission committee, and the first class assembled that fall. "It is not our intention to rebuild Mayo institutions in the image of a medical school," he said on the eve of the school's opening, "but to introduce the process of education of undergraduate medical students into the setting of one of the world's greatest medical centers, where the primary concern is for excellence of care of the individual patient." Noting the small number of students entering Mayo Medical School's first class—a total of forty—Pruitt referred to the Latin inscription above the main entrance of the medical school: *non multa sed bono* (not many, but good). This school, he told the students, "at its inception was dedicated to the purposes of revolution, in the academic spirit uniting faculty and students alike into a professional elite. Together, they cherished an imperative for the humane in an age made rich by technology and science. And this was the covenant of their ordination: that with the eyes of compassion they assessed the brilliance of their technologies, and with the yardstick of the humane they measured the benefactions of their science."

A few months later, on December 18, 1972, medical students and school administrators moved into the remodeled Rochester Public Library, renamed the Mayo Medical School Student Center. Years earlier, Mayo had donated the land to the city. It seemed fitting that Mayo buy the building, now too small for the library's growing requirements. The student-faculty lounge in the new Mayo Medical School Student Center was named for two long-time friends of Mayo, Walter and Kay O'Malley. Their son, Peter O'Malley, president of the Los Angeles Dodgers, attended the dedication of the lounge. (When Walter O'Malley held that title, he moved the Brooklyn Dodgers to Los Angeles after they won their second World Series in 1959. O'Malley's decision was so unpopular with fans that sports writers Pete Hamill and Jack Newfield once listed their top three choices for the worst human beings who ever lived as Hitler, Stalin, and Walter O'Malley!)

second dean of Mayo Medical School

When Raymond Pruitt retired in 1977, I succeeded him as director for education and dean of Mayo Medical School. Since both of us were the sons of clergymen, I quoted Ecclesiastes 9:7 at his retirement dinner: "Go, eat your bread with enjoyment and drink your wine with a merry heart—for God has already approved what you do." As Congressman Albert H. Quie of Minnesota echoed in a letter to me after my appointment as dean: "As you probably know, I have been very interested in the establishment of the Mayo Medical School and supportive of that effort. Everything I have heard about the progress to date has been favorable, due in large part to Pruitt's dedication and excellent direction."

I resolved to continue Pruitt's policy of exposing medical students to patients and their medical problems from the beginning of their training at Mayo. He felt strongly, and so did I, that they would immediately understand the relevance of the medical sciences to the clinical problems encountered in practice. But I altered another decision. Pruitt did not believe Mayo needed anatomists to teach the structure of the body and thus surgeons taught the subject, focusing on the relative importance of different organs in relationship to disease. Not only were surgeons too busy to teach anatomy, but the external review committee deciding whether to continue licensing medical schools told me that Mayo must have a professional anatomist. Years before, anatomists had taught in the Mayo Graduate School, but by this time they had retired and not been replaced. Thus, my first order of business was to find an anatomist. I selected Donald R. Cahill from the University of Miami, who recruited Stephen W. Carmichael from the University of West Virginia. Teaching full-time, the two made the study of anatomy a success much appreciated by students at Mayo.

Pruitt also required each entering student to complete the Minnesota Multiphasic Personality Index as part of the admissions process. I agreed that we should continue its use, but students said the MMPI was an invasion of privacy they could not accept. The associate dean for student affairs agreed, and so we dropped the test. In instructing the admissions committee, however, I followed my predecessor's example: two members conducted separate interviews of prospective students for a broader perspective of the applicants.

The work of the admissions committee was anything but easy, since well over three thousand applicants sought the forty (now forty-two) places in each entering class. The committee reviewed all the applications, then selected about three hundred prospective students to interview. Committee members often found they could quickly determine the exceptional applicants and those who should not be admitted. But it was more difficult to select those between. To help the committee when it really could not decide, I proposed drawing applicants' names from a hat for the available places. Instead of writing a negative letter to those not admitted, we could tell them that our small school could not admit all who were qualified, that we had selected by lottery. Someone voiced the opinion that a lottery would provoke lawyers eager to sue the institution for students approved but not admitted. That may have been a proper concern!

About half the students admitted to Mayo Medical School today are women. The 1996 entering class was 54.7 percent female, the first time women had outnumbered men. The increase in the number of women training side by side with men is a remarkable change from a century ago. Queen Victoria had dismissed "the awful idea of allowing young girls and young men to enter the anatomy dissecting room together, where the young girls would have to study things which could not be named before them." Even soon after I came permanently to the United States, I lectured on my research at the University of Washington in Seattle and I asked how many women were in the current class at the medical school there. The answer was none. At that time in Great Britain and in my own medical school in Belfast, about 20 to 30 percent of all medical students were women. Efforts to recruit qualified women to the Mayo staff had to wait until the number of female medical school graduates increased. Today, the number of women on the Mayo staff continues to increase. The number of minority medical students and staff has also increased. Mayo actively seeks qualified minorities, including Native and African Americans. In 2002, Mayo Medical School was fifteenth among U.S. medical schools ranked by *U.S. News and World Report.*

Mayo's medical school has established an award recognizing distinguished educators. The award helps to highlight the importance that Mayo places on medical education and provides meaningful faculty recognition throughout the institution. In addition, Mayo has created an appointment category for educators who make teaching an important part of their responsibilities at Mayo. Mayo also looks at how medical education faculty members can enhance their skills through electronic education.

who would be a dean?

When I was a dean, I enjoyed learning about the perceived vicissitudes of the duties and responsibilities of the office. For example, Philip Rhodes wrote an article in the *British Medical Journal* in 1977 when he was medical dean at the University of Adelaide in South Australia. "In founding the monastery of Monte Cassino in the sixth century," wrote Rhodes, "[St. Benedict] divided the brotherhood into groups of ten, over whom he set one—the dean. The dictionary gives derivations from *doyen* and the Greek *dekanos,* meaning one set over ten. Nowadays some members of the decanal group might often wish that they had only ten others to deal with."

According to Rhodes, a dean's duties leave little time for research, reading, teaching, practice, or writing. In fact, he declared no one in his or her right mind would seek a post with such innumerable committees and endless chores. "All is supposed to be subject to democratic dispute in which the will of the majority will prevail after listening to the arguments," he wrote "and those in the minority will acquiesce in what their wiser brethren have agreed. How such a jejune belief could come to be accepted by a group of otherwise intelligent persons is beyond comprehension. But that is the way in which medical schools are believed to be run. So the successful dean, if there is any such person, is the one who can keep the level of frustration within acceptable bounds."

Rhodes concluded, "There can be little wonder that the dean's job is impossible. By virtue of the academic system he has no control over his colleagues in the faculty, who will give authority to him only fitfully, often grudgingly, and in a way on which he can never rely. His only resources would seem to be information, persuasion, and some moral authority of varying degree. But to some irrepressible natures with rhinoceros hides, it can be fun."

Several colleagues added their take on what it means to be a dean. One prominent associate at an assembly of deans in the Association of Academic Medical Centers told me that deans can take refuge in a club called "Deans Anonymous": when you have a brilliant idea for a change, you call a certain number and another dean will sit with you until the idea goes away! Another told me about a dean invited to be president of a heavenly university. After he accepted, God informed him that the university had *two* medical schools. The former dean replied, "There must be some mistake. I thought I was in heaven—but I must be in hell!" I heard yet another story about the dean of a medical school whose predecessor left three letters on his desk. With the numbered letters was a note: "Open in this order when you have problems." Soon enough, the new dean encountered his first problem. He opened the first envelope: "Blame the faculty." He blamed the faculty, and things settled down for a while. But soon there was more trouble, so he opened the second envelope: "Blame the students." Once again, things settled down, but trouble reappeared. The third and final letter read: "Write three letters."

Stories about deans may be exceeded only by those about lawyers, but my experience at Mayo was quite different from the stories. Just as with the Mayo Research Committee, I found the Mayo Education Committee an essential sounding board. The members listened carefully, made thoughtful suggestions and appropriate comments, and counseled me on policy. I always found the relationship constructive. The members helped me advance all aspects of Mayo's educational programs. This experience reflects the Mayo principle of full-time salaries, with no bonus system and no profit sharing, which results in little need for "turf protection" seen among some medical groups. The tenure system in place at other academic medical centers, combined with the authority of the department chairs and long years of seniority, makes consensus difficult to achieve. And although an associate alerted me that I should not anticipate much change in salary when I became dean, in truth I spent only part of my time as dean and director of education, and I had sufficient administrative help to accomplish what I needed to do. For the balance, I continued working on research with talented young colleagues from many countries.

I can say from personal experience that educators are fully aware that economists, epidemiologists, psychologists, social planners, and statisticians scrutinize every aspect of life today. As proof, I offer the 131 questionnaires I received in my first year as dean. Such material contributes to what someone has called "paralysis by analysis," a syndrome endemic in our society. The questionnaires sought my views on such topics as the academic frustration syndrome, the hierarchical ambiguity of the dysfunctional status gap between nonphysician health administrators and physician-clinicians, how to measure the medical school learning environment, deviant groups of medical school applicants, and psychiatry and mysticism—not to mention how I might foster increased sensitivity and communication as perceived by the medical student's spouse or other partner!

A dean also frequently receives government publications. One I particularly cherished came from the Bureau of Health Manpower of the Health Resources Administration of the Public Health Service of the Department of Health, Education, and Welfare. It was DHEW Publication No. (HRA) 77–55, *An Empirical Classification of United States Medical Schools by Institutional Dimensions,* prepared by the Association of American Medical Colleges in 1977 under contract number 231-76-0011. From it, I learned that the "non-hierarchical cluster analysis method used in this study was developed by Forgy (1965) and is known as the K-means technique." It continued:

> *Using the number of clusters and cluster centroids specified by the user, each object is assigned to the cluster with the closest centroid. After all objects have been initially assigned to a cluster, new cluster centroids are computed for each cluster based on the objects assigned to the cluster. The distance of each object from each of the cluster centroids is then computed and objects are reassigned, if necessary, to the cluster which now has the closest centroid. After the reassignment of objects, the cluster centroids are recomputed, and a new cycle of computing distances, reassigning schools, and recomputing cluster centroids is begun. . . . Based on the results of the six factor hierarchical cluster analysis, an optimal solution was sought using Forgy's non-hierarchical cluster analysis method. The results of the*

> *hierarchical clustering were used to give an indication of the number of clusters which would represent the schools, and schools were selected as seed points for the non-hierarchical cluster analysis based on the hierarchical clusters. In the hierarchical cluster analysis, one school, the Mayo Medical School, appeared so dissimilar from the other 109 schools that it was not included in further comparisons.*

Unacquainted with the Forgy method, I was reassured by another paragraph: "The Forgy non-hierarchical cluster analysis technique complements the Ward hierarchical method by optimizing the same criterion, the sum of the squared distances of the schools from the cluster centroids, but does not maintain the permanence of cluster membership inherent in the hierarchical methods."

Pretty heavy stuff, to be sure!

While I was dean of Mayo Medical School, the Stanford University School of Medicine tried to recruit me for a similar position. The letter I received in February 1981 from the chair of the search committee said I had been "strongly recommended as a candidate" for dean. The dean would serve also as an associate vice president of the Stanford Medical Center and be chief academic officer of the medical school with responsibility for academic programs. I much appreciated the compliment, but after reviewing my commitments at Mayo and discussing it with Helen and several colleagues, I decided to stay at Mayo.

Many of us from Queen's University became deans of medical schools: two in Australia, at the University of Adelaide (Robert Whelan) and the University of New South Wales in Sydney (William Glover); one in England at the University of Nottingham (David Greenfield); three in succession at Queen's University in Belfast (Ian Roddie, Robin Shanks, and Gary Love); and I at Mayo.

Whelan later became vice chancellor of the University of Western Australia in Perth, then vice chancellor at the University of Liverpool in England. There he received the formal notice that he was selected for knighthood. By long tradition, Queen Elizabeth would touch his shoulder with a sword and say, "Arise, Sir Robert." Alas, Whelan died suddenly before the formal ceremony took place.

David Greenfield, who succeeded Henry Barcroft as chair of the physiology department at Queen's University, subsequently achieved international distinction as a founder of medical schools. The first was in Nottingham, where

Queen Elizabeth named him a Commander of the British Empire. The other two medical schools he founded are in Hong Kong and Qaboos, Oman, where he received the Order of the Sultan of Qaboos.

When my former Belfast colleague, William Glover, retired as dean of the Medical School of New South Wales, I traveled to Sydney to give the formal address at his retirement ceremony at the Royal Sydney Golf Club. I recalled that we had once known Dean Glover as "Darty" because as a child he was always a darter.

In 1986, I also gave a keynote address at the celebrations for the 150th anniversary of Queen's University's medical school. During my deanship, I too extended invitations to distinguished men and women to address Mayo Medical School ceremonies, including annual graduation. One such person was associate justice Harry Andrew Blackmun, a former head of Mayo's legal department whom President Nixon had appointed to the Supreme Court in 1970. "I hope you will have interests beyond the consulting room, the hospital, the operating room, the laboratory, and the medical library," Blackmun told the graduates of 1980. "We all live in a big, unsheltered, complex world. And you are a vital, educated, valuable part of that world. It needs your interest and your participation. You are intelligent human beings, and the world today needs all the intelligence it can find."

Two years later I invited Hanna Gray to speak at the commencement exercises. An eminent historian, Gray was then president of the University of Chicago as well as a public trustee of the Mayo Foundation. She told the 1982 Mayo graduates that many people utter anti-science sentiments "out of the fear of being unable to understand, and therefore to control, what science creates. There is the fear that science by itself will be a runaway force on which people will become dependent, rather than an instrument that people may shape to larger human and social purposes. In that fear is the thought that it would be better not to promote and support discovery but rather to be satisfied to control what we already know, that with new knowledge might come loss of control, that some will take over a new knowledge and make others the servants of it."

A fear of science often leads to a lack of appreciation for discovery and knowledge. "It has been argued over and over again that because knowledge can be abused, it is therefore dangerous," said Gray. "But this view overlooks the simple truth that what is good or evil in the use of knowledge comes from our purposes and motivations in using it and not from the thing itself. The great danger before us is that constraint and the need to find solutions to current problems may lead to short-term resolutions and narrow thinking, and to a kind of hunkering down within our own roles because it looks so complex out there."

Mayo becomes a degree-granting institution

As director for education from 1977 to 1983, I wished to see Mayo become a degree-granting institution, since this would ensure that Mayo's governing bodies would accept the responsibility of guaranteeing the quality of Mayo education programs to outside reviewing bodies. In August 1981 I had the support of the board of governors and that of the board of trustees to explore the possible establishment of Mayo Clinic and Foundation as a degree-granting institution. By this time, Mayo Medical School recognized that its relationship with the University of Minnesota was only a paper transaction. There was no significant interaction between the two institutions. Indeed, we felt it important that our investigators collaborate with colleagues at many institutions.

In May 1982, board of governors chair W. Eugene Mayberry and I met with C. Peter Magrath, president of the University of Minnesota, and Lyle French, vice president for Health Sciences. There was no discussion about the possible benefits of continuing the academic affiliation between Mayo and the university. French said he supported the disaffiliation and that Mayo had demonstrated it was capable of conducting the education programs it had established. President Magrath also had no objection to the separation, but he emphasized that the university would keep the money earlier left it by the Mayo brothers, worth by then more than $5 million.

While such discussions about the endowment fund continued, we at Mayo moved for approval from both the Minnesota Higher Education Coordinating Board and the North Central Association for Mayo to award the medical, doctorate, and master of science degrees. The Mayo master's degree in biomedical sciences was to replace the clinical degree for residents previously offered in affiliation with the University of Minnesota.

Later in 1982, I wrote to Edward S. Petersen, secretary of the American Medical Association's Liaison Committee on Medical Education, that in its first decade the Mayo Medical School was "securely established as an integral part of the Mayo Foundation and Clinic, with enthusiastic support from faculty, students, graduates, and residency program directors." I pointed out that the school had an endowment of more than $50 million, a teaching faculty of 780 physicians and scientists, more than eight hundred residents and postdoctoral resident fellows in graduate programs, an annual patient registration in excess of 250,000, and two affiliated hospitals with eighteen hundred beds—all available for teaching purposes. Funding for research at Mayo amounted to $44 million in 1981, 30 percent of which the Mayo Foundation provided. After summarizing the discussions among all the involved institutions and governing bodies, I requested that Petersen's committee "continue full accreditation of Mayo Medical School and . . . approve the transfer to the board of trustees of Mayo Foundation and the officials of Mayo Medical School the authority to grant the M.D. degree effective with the class to graduate in May 1983."

On December 2, 1982, the Minnesota Higher Education Coordinating Board permitted Mayo Foundation to grant the medical degree and the doctoral degree in the biomedical sciences. The board gave permission at its meeting on April 28, 1983, for Mayo to grant the master's degree in biomedical sciences. On March 30, 1983, the North Central Association had also stated that Mayo was eligible for accreditation as an institution of postsecondary education.

In May 1983, after I had left the post of director for education and dean of the medical school (my successor was Franklin Knox), the University of Minnesota board of regents and the Mayo Foundation board of trustees resolved at separate meetings to recognize the end of the academic affiliation between Mayo and the university effective June 30, 1983.

The road to independence was not without its molehills. One opponent speculated the move was an effort to circumvent a policy requiring admission primarily of state residents. Thus, many Mayo alumni living outside Minnesota might push to get their children into Mayo Medical School. The *Princeton Union-Eagle* declared disappointment "that this has apparently been discussed for a year by the leadership of both institutions without taking the public into their confidence, without public hearings, without any public inputs whatever. There are medical questions about which the lay public cannot presume to have knowledge. But on matters of public policy affecting the training of physicians and carrying on research, we feel the public that foots the bills is entitled to some consideration."

After the meeting in Minneapolis in May 1982, when President Magrath said the university would keep the sixty-six-year-old Mayo endowment, the question of what would become of the money lingered. Again, Stephen F. Keating, chair of the Mayo board of trustees, had a straightforward, efficient way of resolving the matter. Keating eventually worked out an arrangement in which Mayo would receive 62.5 percent of the fund, the university the remaining 37.5 percent. Magrath pledged a large part of the university's share to endow a faculty chair in public health.

Soon after it became apparent that Mayo Medical School would receive approval for granting degrees independent of the University of Minnesota, I asked James R. McPherson, dean for academic affairs, to recommend colors and a design for a graduation hood. "As I thought about colors," McPherson wrote in response, "my mind skipped about to my own alma mater, team colors, a huge variety of colors displayed in catalogues, and finally to a phrase 'there are as many opinions as there are men.' I needed to have some credible basis for whatever we chose, and it clearly should be different from the University of Minnesota colors."

Because his own university colors were "uninspiring," McPherson turned to the flag of the state of Minnesota, "dominated by blue and gold, the city of Rochester flag similarly containing much blue with gold trim." Would other members of the education committee find blue and gold acceptable as the Mayo colors? After a spirited discussion, Robert R. Hattery (later chair of the board of governors) said he loved the colors McPherson proposed—they were the colors of his wife's high school!

With such an endorsement, the committee selected green, blue, and gold, and the students ascending the podium in 1983 to receive Mayo medical degrees thus became the first class to assume the new Mayo hood. The event truly celebrated the formal recognition by state and national accrediting bodies of Mayo Medical School's coming of age.

Today, both the Mayo Foundation and the University of Minnesota regard the history of Mayo's independence after so long an association with the university not so much as a disaffiliation but as a recognition of two independent institutions. Each contributes to the biomedical sciences through education and research, and each participates in an interchange that benefits both, as well as the citizens of Minnesota and the world.

Mayo's educational programs

Today, the Mayo Graduate School of Medicine is one of the world's largest graduate education centers. In 1930, the Mayo Graduate School trained 285 medical residents, 14 percent of the total then in training in the United States. As of 2001, the number of residents and clinical fellows trained at Mayo was 1,219—1,036 at Rochester, 99 at Jacksonville, and 84 at Scottsdale.

(So many others were in training elsewhere in the United States by then that the percentage of the national total trained by Mayo was 1 percent, considerably less than in 1930.) Some of those in training in Rochester also have rotations at Mayo centers in Jacksonville, Florida, and Scottsdale, Arizona.

In addition to those studying for medical degrees—forty-two per class—Mayo admits six students per year for the combined medical and doctoral degree, a six-year program. Areas of study are biochemistry, biomedical engineering, immunology, molecular neuroscience, molecular pharmacology, and tumor biology.

The Mayo School of Health Sciences enrolls approximately 360 students annually in twenty-six allied health programs. More than 310 courses are offered each year to various medical professionals attending the Mayo School of Continuing Medical Education programs.

The Mayo master's degree program provides a discipline for those who wish an experience in research to become better informed and more critical clinical consultants. Today, the counsel of Mayo Foundation's first chair, Louis B. Wilson, seems more relevant than ever: "The fixed graduate school requirement of attempted research by every member of its student body has been accepted by Mayo Foundation because it believes that everyone competent to act as a consultant in a special field of medicine should have enough experience in controlled research . . . to evaluate the research work of others and to conduct investigations . . . in a scientific manner."

Wilson did not intend to confine research to studies in the laboratory but to include any study of new knowledge of value to medicine. In setting forth as an independent degree-granting body, Mayo Clinic and Foundation affirmed its faith in the concept that the best medical care depends on the interdependence of practice, education, and research. "Our organization concerns sick people, and it is necessary to have a liberal attitude toward those who are responsible for the care of the patient and to see that necessary rules and regulations do not needlessly interfere with the initiative of members of the staff," said Will Mayo in 1932.

Today, recognizing the importance of understanding the religious beliefs of its patients, Mayo Medical School (like other medical schools) has organized a Spirituality and Healthcare Lecture Series. The series surveys spiritual perspectives and their impact on health, illness, and the dying process among different faiths, including Animism, Christianity, Eastern religions, Islam, Judaism, and Native American traditions.

Mayo Foundation House

Mayo Foundation House symbolizes the Mayo principle of continuing medical education. Once the home of Will and Hattie Mayo, who wanted their house to be a place of hospitality for visiting physicians and others, the forty-seven-room, twenty-four-thousand-square-foot Tudor-style house was completed in 1918. Built on the block where city pioneer George Head's brick home once stood, the castlelike stone house sits close to downtown Rochester. The Minnesota architectural firm of Ellerbe included a tower at Dr. Will's request. His parents' home had a similar tower where his mother could view the heavens with a telescope.

With its spacious grounds and gardens, the home quickly became a social center where the Mayos entertained many dignitaries. When the Mayos moved to a smaller house on the grounds in 1938 (now called Damon House, in honor of Hattie Damon Mayo), they donated the house to the Mayo Foundation for use as a "place where men and women of medicine exchange ideas for the good of mankind."

Much of the original decor of Mayo Foundation House remains to provide a functional yet gracious setting for lectures, seminars, dinner meetings, and other educational activities. Balfour Hall, named for surgeon Donald C. Balfour, one of the clinic's original five partners, is a spacious meeting room on the third floor. Hanging above the fireplace is a fine portrait of the Mayo brothers by John C. Johansen. After the Mayos gave the house to Mayo Foundation, the walls of Balfour Hall were paneled in dark New England oak with escutcheons representing the medical schools of the Mayo staff members in 1938. Among them is my own school, Queen's University of Belfast, also the alma mater of James W. Kernohan, head of Mayo's surgical pathology section. Members of the Kernohan family still lived at that time in County Antrim, Northern Ireland, and my brother Fred was their physician.

In the living room of Mayo Foundation House is the "lost portrait" by the Norwegian-born artist Brynjulf Strandenes. The portrait features the Mayo brothers in an operating room, their parents in the background looking on. Other figures in the portrait are Will Mayo's son-in-law, Waltman Walters, and his scrub nurse, Sister Joseph, as well as John S. Lundy, founder of the Mayo Department of Anesthesiology. The lost portrait acquired its name in an interesting fashion. Strandenes immigrated to the United States in 1914 after working as an artist and cartoonist for an Oslo newspaper. During his most productive years, the 1920s and 1930s, Strandenes executed portraits of prominent people, including King Haakon VII of Norway and the opera singer Kirsten Flagstad (that portrait later hung in the Metropolitan Opera

House in New York). After Strandenes became a close friend of Charles and Edith Mayo, he painted a historical Mayo family portrait using an operating-room setting. The painting never entirely satisfied the artist, however. Strandenes, who experienced periods of depression, once nearly destroyed it with an ice pick. After suffering a massive stroke, Strandenes gave the restored painting in June 1951 to a friend, surgeon Kaare K. Nygaard, who trained at the Mayo Clinic during the early 1930s. Nearly two decades after Strandenes died in 1953, Nygaard donated the portrait in 1971 to Mayo Foundation House.

During my years as dean, I proposed that we recognize outstanding members of the Mayo Alumni Association. Mayo conferred its first Distinguished Alumnus Awards in 1981. The staff recommends candidates, and the Division of Education selects those who will receive the awards. Reflecting the international character of the Mayo Graduate School of Medicine, many of the recipients have been Mayo alumni from outside the United States who later achieved prominence in medicine in their own countries. Their successes provide a special recognition of Mayo in many countries. By 2002, the number of graduate-school alumni was more than fifteen thousand. I was both surprised and honored to receive the Distinguished Alumnus Award in 1985.

guest lectures here and abroad

Since completing my terms as Mayo dean and director for education in 1983, I have remained keenly interested in medical education. Invited to lecture at many medical schools, I always used these occasions to learn about others' experiences with medical education. The schools include the University of Wisconsin at Milwaukee (Rieck Memorial Lecture), the University of Southern California (Nathanson Memorial Lecture), the University of California Medical School at San Francisco, Harvard (Grand Rounds), and the University of Minnesota (Visiting Professor). Outside the United States the schools were St. Thomas's Hospital Medical School in London (Sherrington Lecture), University of Nottingham (George Cecil Clarke Lecture), the University of Alberta in Edmonton, Canada, the medical school in Leiden, Holland (Einthoven Lecture), Tel Aviv University, Israel (the first Raymond and Beverly Sackler Distinguished Lecture in Medicine), and the University of Auckland (New Zealand).

My trip to Auckland involved a pleasant stay over a period of some weeks in 1994. The roots of this story go back to 1959, when I developed a friendship with John D. Sinclair, who was at the Mayo Clinic in 1959 and 1960 on a postdoctoral fellowship from the U.S. Public Health Service. He had earned his medical degree at the University of New Zealand in 1950 and had done postdoctoral training in New Zealand, the United Kingdom, and Scandinavia. At Mayo, he worked in the Department of Physiology and Biophysics with Earl Wood. As a member of the department, I soon came to know John and his wife, Patricia, an accomplished potter. After the Sinclairs returned to New Zealand, John became professor of physiology in the University of Auckland School of Medicine in 1968. He chaired the department until 1983, then was subdean for human biology from 1984 until 1986. He chaired the department again from 1991 to 1993.

In Sinclair's honor, Paul McNeil Hill organized an international symposium—"Exercise: The Physiological Challenge"—at the University of Auckland in 1992. Hill, a member of the physiology department at the university and a fellow Irishman, invited me to attend. I recommended that Jere Mitchell of the University of Texas, an internationally known researcher on exercise, join me at the meeting in Auckland. Together we discussed factors controlling the circulation in exercise.

Soon after the 1992 symposium, I received a second invitation from Hill, who was in charge of teaching physiology to medical students and candidates for the bachelor of science degree. This time the invitation was to spend June and July 1994 at the Auckland medical school giving lectures on the cardiovascular system. I was to give four lectures each week, Monday through Thursday, to the medical students and six weeks of lectures to the bachelor of science candidates. This meant I would be free from Thursday afternoons to Sunday evenings to explore New Zealand with my wife.

Our journey from Rochester to Auckland was not without incident. We arrived in Los Angeles from Minneapolis–St. Paul and were waiting to board the plane for Auckland when I heard my name called. At the counter, I learned that during the transfer of our bags from Northwest Airlines to New Zealand Air, a van had run over one of our bags. All of the slides for my lectures were in one of those bags! A short time later, the bags arrived at the New Zealand counter, and we found the very damaged bag, bound with plastic.

We continued on to New Zealand, where Hill met us at the Auckland airport. I later enjoyed meeting and working with the students and found them the equal of the students I had taught at the medical schools of Queen's and Mayo. On one occasion I mentioned to them that in America the initials "TGIF" stand for "Thank God It's Friday." In response, they said they used a similar term in New Zealand, POETS, which means "Piss Off Early, Tomorrow's Saturday!"

Rochester Epidemiology Project

I cannot discuss medical education at Mayo without mentioning Leonard T. Kurland, who established the clinic in Rochester as a premier center of epidemiological studies. As a neurological fellow at Mayo Clinic in the 1950s, Kurland (who earned his medical degree from the University of Maryland, his master's in public health from Harvard, and his doctorate in public health from Johns Hopkins) perceived the significance of the medical records system devised by Henry Plummer. After joining the Mayo staff, Kurland introduced the Rochester Epidemiology Project in 1966. This medical-records linkage system has made Olmsted County one of the few places in the world with a historic and continuing record of the occurrence and course of disease.

From its beginnings, the Mayo Clinic has provided medical care for much of the population of Rochester (the county seat) and Olmsted County. Its medical records give a complete history of medical care from birth to death, often to autopsy. Such data is invaluable to epidemiologists. In 1976, for example, there was a national program of immunization against the swine-flu strain of influenza, which was similar to the strain that killed as many as twenty-one million people during the worldwide influenza pandemic of 1918–1919. The swine flu did not develop as a killer strain, but health authorities soon began to note among those who had been inoculated (fifty million Americans in ten weeks) a relatively large number of patients diagnosed with Guillain-Barré syndrome, a rare neuromuscular disorder. Was this to be expected or something of concern? After examining the rate of the syndrome in the population of Olmsted County, Mayo epidemiologists concluded that recipients of the swine-flu vaccine were developing Guillain-Barré syndrome at a rate several times normal. As a result, the national immunization ended.

Based on Olmsted County health and medical records, the Institute of Medicine of the National Academy of Sciences concluded in a June 1999 report that there was insufficient evidence to support an association of silicone breast implants with defined connective tissue disease. Without evidence of an association, the report, "Safety of Silicone Breast Implants," concluded there is "no justification for the use of resources in further epidemiological exploration of such an association."

Matters concerning Mayo's patients and the clinic's medical practice were as much a focus for me as my research and education responsibilities during the 1960s, 1970s, and 1980s. Decisions about such matters were made through a powerful entity of which I was a member for fourteen years: the Mayo board of governors.

5

governing Mayo's practice

Mayo's three-part mission of research, education, and practice mirrored the focus of my administrative assignments at the clinic. Eight years as director for research and six years as director for education had overlapped and intertwined with my tenure on Mayo's board of governors, the chief decision-making body of the clinic. As a member of the board from 1966 to 1980, I participated firsthand in the decisions concerning medical practice made and implemented at Mayo, and I came to appreciate the observation that the factor distinguishing successful organizations from others is often the ability to change.

During those fourteen years, my colleagues and I saw nothing but change. We approved the expansion of facilities for patient care, including a ten-story addition to the Mayo Building, as well as the construction of the Baldwin Building for Community Medicine, the Guggenheim Research Building, and the Conrad N. Hilton Building for Laboratory Medicine. We launched the Department of Internal Medicine and the Division of Hypertension, and laid the groundwork for building the Gonda Vascular Center. We even explored a system of electronic medical-recordkeeping that was later implemented in the 1990s.

But the groundbreakings with the greatest impact on the Mayo Clinic's growth in patient care came not in Rochester, Minnesota, but in Jacksonville, Florida, and Scottsdale, Arizona. Toward the end of my term on the board, we began considering possibilities for new Mayo Clinic sites in those two cities. Within seven years, Mayo Clinic Jacksonville and Mayo Clinic Scottsdale had opened – truly crowning achievements of the Mayo board of governors.

Mayo board of governors

Nine years after joining the Mayo staff, I began my service on the board of governors, which had created the position to which I was elected on November 21, 1966, thus increasing its number of medical members from nine to ten. I served on the board until 1980. After my first meeting, Edward Henderson, a senior member, took me aside to welcome me and offer his support. He advised me to be an active participant, to say my piece, and not to be subservient to more senior members. Henderson's father had founded the Department of Orthopedic Surgery and established its success. Since he was a member of what we called "the royal family"—a descendant of the first five associates of the Mayo brothers—I appreciated Henderson's advice.

The board of governors selects committee members with input from their colleagues on the staff. Those who serve are the best qualified, without regard to seniority or other considerations. Appointment to the now twelve-member board of governors requires ratification of the entire Mayo staff. Members serve staggered four-year terms, and the board elects its own officers each year. Nominations to the board come from informal consultation with a large segment of clinic leadership, as well as with officers and councilors of the staff. Councilors are elected at the annual staff meeting. While they have no official role in governance or administration, councilors advise the board about staff views and recommendations. Board officers and councilors together organize and conduct regular staff meetings.

Rather than rely on a hierarchy of individuals with authority to make unilateral decisions, Mayo employs a collaborative system in which interdependent committees with broad representation work together with the governing boards to reach decisions. The Mayos and their partners established the principle that the medical and scientific staff would make governing decisions for Mayo's future in education, research, and medical practice. Three key committees thus report to the board: medical practice, education, and research. Mayo committees are the vehicles through which physicians and administrators work together to direct the overall management of the institution, plan for the future, and ensure that the principles established by our founders are upheld. Each committee includes a voting nonmedical administrator who provides information and writes the minutes, but the great majority are from the medical and scientific staffs. While the medical and scientific staffs are responsible for key decisions, they consider the advice and wisdom of their administrative colleagues. As with all other Mayo committees, the board selects the medical members of the three major committees with input from the staff on the basis of who is best qualified, without regard to seniority.

One long-standing principle is that medical members, including governors and trustees, continue to carry out their clinical and research duties while governing. Maintaining their professional practices keeps the medical members in touch with colleagues and everyday operations and enables them to return full-time to their other responsibilities when they complete their board service. Staff members also are more likely to accept decisions made by their own working colleagues than by full-time administrators or colleagues no longer on the front line.

In the first two decades of my career at Mayo, the board of governors followed another collaborative principle: whenever a committee acted on a request, a key member (often the chair) would visit the originator to explain the committee's action. If the decision were negative, the proponent would have an opportunity to appear before the committee. While this policy was time-consuming, we members of the board recognized its importance in maintaining good relations with our colleagues. The social outcome of a personal visit exceeded the more efficient but less satisfactory explanation of a printed statement dictated by the committee secretary. As the size of Mayo's staff increased, however, it became more difficult to maintain this policy.

Even though I was a researcher, I was directly involved in patient care. And although medicine is serious business, I have always enjoyed sharing humorous stories about medical practice. Chuck Mayo, who joined the staff as a surgeon in the 1930s, is the subject of many such anecdotes. Once, Dr. Chuck spoke with a patient without having looked carefully at her hospital chart. "If we could just get your bowel movements straightened out, you would be in good condition," he said to her with encouragement. "But I have a good, normal bowel movement every day," replied the perplexed patient. Thinking quickly, he responded, "Ah, yes! But the bowel movement you had today was a day late—you *should* have had it yesterday!"

Another favorite story concerns the patient who confided to his doctor, "I know what's wrong with me. The Holy Ghost told me." Doctor: "Then why did you come to the Mayo Clinic?" Patient: "I wanted a second opinion." Yet another involves the concerns of a colleague at Mayo treating a member of the Mafia. An armed bodyguard always accompanied the patient, even during medical examinations. "Mainly I was fearful that I'd be dropped in a nearby lake with my feet in cement if he died under my care!" the physician commented.

But I took my responsibilities for Mayo's medical practice as seriously as I had taken those in research and education, and upon my election to the board I was pleased to receive several letters of congratulations and encouragement from colleagues. One letter was from Alexander Albert of the Section of Endocrine Research, who wrote the first funding application that the Mayo Clinic submitted to the National Institutes of Health. "I've heard nothing but praise and admiration for your efforts," Albert wrote me. "This comes from all quarters, and sometimes from unexpected (at least to me) sources. Coupled with this is an equal admiration for your personality, your integrity, and courage with which you approach problems. Do persevere!"

the Mayo Building

During my fourteen-year service on the board of governors, Mayo constructed several major buildings and additions to provide space for its growing needs. By 1966, the Mayo Building was being used to capacity; the clinic needed more space. A multispecialty group of physicians working in the pattern conceived by the Mayos and Henry Plummer had designed the Mayo Building to facilitate medical care. (Plummer, who joined the clinic staff in 1901 and devised Mayo's revolutionary medical records dossier system, was second only to the Mayos in shaping the practice we know today.) The Mayo Building opened in 1955 to serve the rapid increase in patient visits following World War II. Studies in 1948 and 1949 had showed that twenty-five thousand to fifty thousand patients annually failed to get appointments because of the high demand for Mayo services.

The exterior of the Mayo Building, which took the shape of a Greek cross, is covered with white and gray Georgia marble. An innovative series of decorative murals, *Mirror to Man,* graces the walls of the central waiting rooms on each floor. The Croatian-born sculptor Ivan Mestrovic created a striking outside addition, *Man and Freedom.* Unveiled in 1954, this twenty-eight-foot, three-ton sculpture, its arms spread gracefully in a posture of supplication, was mounted on the north wall of the building. ("This looks like a man who has just received his account for medical services rendered!" a patient once told me.) The statue was removed for restoration in 2000 and since reinstalled on the same wall as a component in the atrium of the new Gonda Building, visible from both outside and inside.

When the Mayo Building first opened, Chuck Mayo complained that the glass panes on the door of his new sixth-floor offices limited his privacy. He wanted offices that would allow him to enjoy an occasional nap after returning from the surgical theater. When his complaint went unheeded, he declared that some people will accept anything architects give them, no matter how dumb—and taped a large picture of the nude Lili St. Cyr over the glass in the door. A few days later he learned he could have a solid wood door if he promised to remove the picture.

By the time I joined the board, it was planning a ten-story addition to the Mayo Building, which was completed in 1969. I took the lead (perhaps my Irish heritage explains it) in the board's decision not to have a floor labeled thirteen, considered by some superstitious patients and even some doctors as a sign of bad luck. Thus, Orthopedics is on the floor labeled fourteen.

As was Mayo's custom, the board of governors asked the orthopedists to work with the architects in planning the department's new digs. This ensured few complaints after completion. We commissioned Thomas Payette, who had a small architectural firm in Massachusetts, to plan the space. According to administrator Robert Roesler, Payette believed that a waiting room had to have an outside window or a series of outside windows. He would not consider locating the waiting rooms adjacent to reception desks and near patient examining rooms, as was typical for other floors of the Mayo Building. Several of us tried to convince him that patients would not look out the window but instead, hoping to hear their name called at any minute, would watch what was going on behind the desk. Payette also believed that chairs in the waiting room should sit in conversational groupings. His design incorporated examining rooms with flexible uses that accommodated the changes in patient mix over the years.

The clinic also commissioned Payette to study the main concourse of the Mayo Building and to make the space feel warmer and less austere. The original concept of the concourse was that it was to be just that: a circulation space, not a waiting room. Here patients register and get information before going to medical appointments on upper floors (and where they return to settle their expenses). Earlier, there had been no place for patients to sit or relax between appointments. Upon Payette's advice, an advisory group, which I chaired, proposed making the central concourse into a waiting space. One administrative colleague—who wished to install a water fountain there—complained no one would see anything but the crotches of people slouching in the chairs! Nonetheless, the seating is there, and I have not observed any need for concern.

The Mayo Building taught us the benefits of completing the first half of what would become tall buildings when first we needed space, and adding the second half when need arose again. One problem with this approach is matching the exterior of an addition to the lower half. For the Mayo Building, we bought enough of the quarry to ensure the proper match in the future.

Harwick Building and Plaza

When it opened in 1960, the Harwick Building was on the edge of the Mayo Clinic campus. As time went on and land-use studies indicated that future construction of buildings should take place south and west of Harwick, its design came into question. Originally intended as a warehouse accommodating thousands of retained x-ray films and medical records, the Harwick Building allowed Epidemiology and Medical Statistics close proximity to records on its first floor.

The building was simple and functional but had little distinction. Its name honored the first chief administrator at Mayo, Harry J. Harwick, who joined the clinic in 1908. Recognizing the benefits of community foundations, he formed a committee of civic leaders in the 1940s to establish such a foundation in Rochester. The Mayo Foundation gave the first gift—$50,000—in 1944.

With the need for a computer center at Mayo came the second stage of the Harwick Building, an eight-story expansion in 1963. Epidemiology and Medical Statistics moved to an upper floor, and the offices of the educational functions of the Mayo Foundation located on the seventh floor. The Mayo Clinic cafeteria moved to the main floor, seminar rooms to the second.

In addition to more space, the expansion offered Mayo the opportunity to improve the building's design. A trustee of the Mayo Foundation, J. Irwin Miller, CEO of Cummings Engineering in Columbus, Indiana, suggested hiring a small Chicago architectural firm, Harry Weese Associates. After reviewing the firm's credentials, the board commissioned Weese to design the Harwick expansion. The architects added windows to the north, south, and west sides and extended the underground walkway to the new building.

I had a particular interest in developing green space downtown, so with expansion of the Harwick Building, Mayo developed Harwick Plaza, a half-acre green area just south of the new structure and north of the Medical Sciences Building. While Harwick Plaza was under construction, the Goulandris family of Athens, Greece, made a serendipitous gift of an imposing bronze for the site. The bronze is the fifteen-foot-high *Four Square Walk-Through* by the English artist Barbara Hepworth. The Goulandris family contributed the Hepworth piece as a memorial to Constantine P. Goulandris, a senior member of the shipping family.

I proposed closing a street that once lay in front of the Medical Sciences Building, abutting Harwick Plaza. I seldom if ever saw a motor vehicle use the street. W. Eugene Mayberry, then chair of the board of governors, supported my idea to convert the street into a green area adjoining the plaza. When we applied to the city for permission to do so, a nearby hotel, though not on that street, maintained that closing the street would limit access to the hotel. We responded with statistics on automobile use of the street, which was minimal. The data convinced the city authorities, who permitted the closing. This green area joined Harwick Plaza to create an attractive park on the campus. Benches provide a place for passersby to relax, enjoy the surroundings, and eat lunch in the spring, summer, and fall.

Baldwin Building

In 1979 we dedicated the Baldwin Building for Community Medicine, named in honor of Jesse and Fern Baldwin of Kearney, Nebraska, for their $5 million endowment to the Mayo Foundation for medical education and research. The Baldwins, founders of the J. A. Baldwin Manufacturing Company, a maker of automotive oil and other filters, were Mayo patients over forty-six years. Just as with the Mayo Building, we completed an addition ten years after Baldwin opened, to provide the needed space with three more floors.

The Baldwin Building was dedicated to the day-to-day and continuing health care needs of Rochester and Olmsted County residents. Its community-oriented medical services include the Divisions of Community Internal Medicine, Acute Illness, Obstetrics, and Community Pediatrics. The building contains a patient education area and educational facilities for Mayo's residents and students of community medicine.

Conrad N. Hilton Building for Laboratory Medicine

When I joined the board of governors in 1966, Mayo's clinical diagnostic laboratories were physically separate. The time had come to coordinate and integrate them. The board had a policy of buying property and land adjacent to the Mayo campus to ensure space for growth. As a result, it was able to coordinate and integrate all of Laboratory Medicine into one building and connect it with the Guggenheim Research Building. This move assisted interaction between the researchers and those designing and developing new tests and procedures in the Conrad N. Hilton Building for Laboratory Medicine, whose name honored the founder of the Hilton Hotel chain.

The completion of the Hilton and Guggenheim Buildings in 1974 represented major additions to the clinic complex in downtown Rochester. Meanwhile, the board of governors appointed W. Eugene Mayberry chair of the new Department of Laboratory Medicine and Pathology. A member of the Mayo Section of Endocrine Research, Mayberry also joined the board, succeeding Emmerson Ward as chair in 1976. At the dedication of the Hilton Building on October 18, 1974, Mayberry called it "unique . . . as a diagnostic center," noting that its design "allows efficiency and economy of operation consistent with providing the highest quality of patient care possible." Thousands of procedures take place in the building every day, millions of diagnostic tests every year. Its laboratories offer full diagnostic services to hospitals and clinics within a one-hundred-mile radius of Rochester.

Through a reference laboratory service, Mayo also analyzes specimens received from referring physicians not just throughout the United States, but throughout the world. This service is centered in the new Vincent A. and Toni Stabile Building, just across the street from the Hilton Building. The Stabile Building was constructed with a major gift from the Madeline C. Stabile Foundation of Verona, New Jersey. Madeline Stabile was vice president of her family's business, Industrial Retaining Ring Company; her family formed the foundation shortly after her death in 1996. The building, which is named for Madeline Stabile's brother and sister, houses a wide range of activities that support Mayo's laboratories, as well as several educational initiatives. Here, three hundred to five hundred specimens per day are referred to 112 different laboratories operating twenty-four hours a day, seven days a week. The reference laboratory makes some sixty thousand phone calls a month to deliver critical and alert values to physicians.

The board invited Alistair Cooke to be the keynote speaker at the dedication of the Hilton and Guggenheim Buildings in 1974. Known for his *Letter from America* radio broadcast to Great Britain during World War II, Cooke wrote numerous books, including *Alistair Cooke's America* and *The Americans: Fifty Letters from America on Our Life and Times.* He addressed a large audience in the reception area for patients in the subway of the Hilton Building, thanking the Murry and Leonie Guggenheim Foundation and Edmond Guggenheim and Conrad Hilton for their philanthropy.

Henry Barcroft, my chief at Queen's University, attended the dedication as a trustee of the Henry Wellcome Foundation. During the reception following the dedication, I introduced Dr. Barcroft and his wife, Biddy, to Cooke—who talked incessantly. After listening for some time, Biddy (who also liked to talk) interrupted: "Mr. Cooke, do you know Ruth Draper?" She referred to a well-known English stage personality of the 1920s through the 1940s who played all the parts, talking nonstop. Cooke got the message at once, saying, "I see what you mean!"

To make room for the Hilton Building, Mayo demolished the old wooden building housing the Wilson Club from 1934 to 1970. The club took its name from Louis B. Wilson, the pathologist described as the "first director of laboratories" at Mayo. He was also the first director of the Mayo Graduate School of Medicine. The Wilson Club, a favorite meeting place for Mayo fellows, had a number of bedrooms for single males and made meals available to all fellows. During 1953 and 1954, when I was a research assistant in the Section of Physiology, I enjoyed spending time there and meeting many of its patrons. All of us were sorry to say good-bye to the Wilson Club.

Michael B. O'Sullivan succeeded Mayberry as chair of the Department of Laboratory Medicine and Pathology in 1975. A specialist in pathology and laboratory medicine, O'Sullivan used his administrative and organizational vision to combine Laboratory Medicine and Pathology into a single department and to develop Mayo Medical Laboratories. He established Mayo's thriving international medical reference laboratory and Mayo Medical Ventures, the health-information and technology transfer arm of the clinic. Both generate income for the benefit of research and education. O'Sullivan also led the development of the regional Mayo Health System in Minnesota, Wisconsin, and Iowa, which now includes almost four hundred physicians and eight hospitals in forty-two communities. He served on the board of governors and the foundation's board of trustees and was president of the Academy of Clinical Laboratory Physicians and Scientists. In 1997 he became chair of the board of governors of Mayo Clinic Scottsdale.

department of internal medicine

In 1966, an external reviewing body placed Mayo's program in internal medicine on probation, citing a lack of defined overall integration of responsibility among sections for graduate medical education programs. In response, the board of governors created the Department of Internal Medicine to coordinate the activities of the growing medical specialties. Richard Reitemeier, a distinguished Mayo gastroenterologist, became chair of this large new department in 1967. The external reviewing body quickly approved our program. With increasing recognition of the importance of integrating practice, education, and research to patient care, we established research units in many of the medical divisions.

Now Internal Medicine includes previously independent sections, or "divisions." Each division takes the title of its specialty plus "Internal Medicine"—thus, the Division of Hematology and Internal Medicine. This naming method indicates the expectation that members of a specialty see patients with problems treated by the specialty and act as general internists as well. The complexities of these specialties become greater over time. Nowadays, consultants spend more and more of their time in their specialties, and the time available for them to act as general internists declines.

Beyond the medical specialties, the Department of Internal Medicine includes the Divisions of Community Internal Medicine and General Internal Medicine. Patients seen in Community Internal Medicine, which started as the L. A. Smith Section in the early 1950s (after the physician who was its first chair), come from the surrounding area of Olmsted County. General Internal Medicine focuses on the medical needs of patients living in the thirty-three counties of southeastern Minnesota and northeastern Iowa. This division serves as an access point for patients seeking appointments at Mayo directly or for patients referred by physicians in the area. More recently, Mayo has established the Mayo Family Clinic Northwest in Rochester.

family medicine

Considering the idea of establishing a practice of family medicine elicited clinicians' concern that some patients might not have access to specialists. The experience of the Department of Internal Medicine, however, satisfied those concerns, and so the board of governors established within it the Division of Family Medicine in 1976. A longtime consultant in cardiovascular diseases, Guy Daugherty, became its temporary chair.

In hiring a permanent chair, those responsible for the medical school wanted someone who would broaden the base of teaching programs and clinical experiences of students. As dean, I had persuaded Robert Avant to take the job in 1977. A well-known family specialist from North Memorial Hospital in Minneapolis, Avant often consulted colleagues in the Mayo medical specialties as was appropriate, gaining their respect. He recruited outstanding colleagues to Mayo as well. Because of his reputation and actions, the Minnesota Academy of Family Medicine approved the family medicine program and expressed increased confidence in Mayo's satellite clinics in Kasson, Plainview, and Zumbrota in southeast Minnesota. Today, Mayo enrolls eight residents each year in its three-year family medicine program.

In recruiting Avant (who later became executive director of Mayo Clinic Jacksonville), the board of governors assured him he could change the Division of Family Medicine, within the Department of Internal Medicine, into a separate department, if he thought this advantageous. He later decided that the division should be separate, so Mayo moved the

Department of Family Medicine in 1977 to the new Baldwin Building.

insurance and medical records

The board of governors often addressed the issue of medical insurance during my years of service. For example, medical insurers had long insisted they would not pay expenses without the patient being admitted to a hospital. Mayo has an equally long-standing principle that every patient receive as much care as possible outside the hospital. The reason is simple: to avoid needless expense. Why should a patient be admitted to a hospital for laboratory and other procedures that can be done more efficiently (and for considerably less cost) at an outpatient clinic? Mayo adopted this principle in its early years, when the top two floors of the Kahler Hotel, adjacent to the clinic, were a hospital. Patients could stay in the lower floors while undergoing tests at the clinic and move to the "high-rent district" on the upper floors as necessary. Despite the best efforts of many Mayo representatives over many long years, insurance companies ignored the obvious logic of this approach.

An incident at my own institution demonstrated that bureaucracy often trumps common sense. The day after a surgical colleague performed a pneumonectomy on a patient with cancer of the lung, he received a telephone call from a representative of an insurance company asking why the patient was still in the hospital. "Because I operated on him," replied the surgeon. The insurance representative asked, "What did you do?" The surgeon answered, then asked: "Do you know what a pneumonectomy is?" "No, I don't," replied the caller, "but it is not on my list of procedures approved for hospitalization." Listening to the conversation, a resident nudged the surgeon: "Tell him it is constipation." The surgeon took his suggestion—to which the insurance agent responded brightly, "Constipation—no problem! That's on my list. He can stay in the hospital."

In the 1960s Lockheed Missiles and Space Corporation had a medical information division endeavoring to set up a commercial hospital-information system. After I joined the board of governors in 1966, Mayo invited the Lockheed unit to work with six physicians on such a system. The physicians spent 50 percent of their time on the project.

Lockheed suggested that Mayo implement an electronic laboratory reporting system and a central appointment desk, *without* including patient medical records in the system at that time. The board of governors authorized a cost-benefit analysis of the proposal, which concluded it was too expensive. Mayo ended the relationship with Lockheed after eighteen months, but the medical records system worked out by the physicians became the basis of the system later adopted at Mayo. In 1993, development of the electronic system for new patient records began.

North Central Cancer Treatment Group

In 1972, as director for research, I met Secretary of Health, Education, and Welfare Elliot L. Richardson at a lunch at the Mayo Clinic. "I was most interested to hear about Mayo's programs and research activities," he wrote later. "I came away with a strong impression of Mayo's unique spirit and tremendous dedication to the goal of improved medical care for the people of this nation."

As an example of this, Frank Rauscher Jr., director of the National Cancer Institute in Washington, reported at a news conference in November 1973 that Mayo had been designated a regional comprehensive cancer center, the ninth of fifteen centers so-named in the nation. Mayo had just introduced the first CT scanner (computed tomography—based on transmitting x-rays) in North America, a vital tool for diagnosing and treating cancer. Mayo was treating more cancer patients than any other medical center in the United States. Rauscher reported that the NCI had pumped about $2 million into Mayo's cancer program.

When Richard Reitemeier left his post as director of Mayo's oncology program to become chair of the newly established Department of Internal Medicine in 1967, the board of governors named David Carr as interim director of the Mayo Cancer Center. But the governors were undecided as to who should be the permanent director. I convinced them that Charles Moertel—who with Reitemeier had started the Mayo oncology program—had demonstrated his ability to develop the necessary clinical, educational, and research programs in this important medical specialty. Internationally known for his clinical investigation of gastrointestinal cancer, Moertel had published more than three hundred manuscripts. The board approved his appointment, and under his leadership the NIH approved Mayo as a comprehensive cancer center. Moertel served as director until 1986, when John Kovach succeeded him.

In 1977 physicians from the Mayo Clinic and other medical institutions in the north central United States developed the North Central Cancer Treatment Group. The purpose was to bring promising new cancer treatments to communities where people live and receive most of their medical care. By the year 2000, this group had treated more than fifty thousand patients. The NIH renewed its funding for cancer research at the Mayo Clinic in 1998 under the leadership of Franklyn Prendergast (appointed Mayo Cancer Center director in 1994) and again named Mayo a comprehensive center, its highest status. The NIH also awarded the center $14.8 million over the following five years.

taking Mayo outside Minnesota

One of the most important discussions of the boards of governors and trustees concerned the pros and cons of developing Mayo medical centers outside Minnesota and its four surrounding states—maybe even outside the United States. I recall one debate on the opportunities for such a center in Luxembourg and another in Guam (suggested in 1973 by the Catholic bishop of Guam during a visit). We took no action on either.

Iran was another possible location. In the last years of Shah Mohammed Reza Pahlevi's reign, there was discussion that Mayo might assist in the construction and staffing of a children's hospital in Teheran. The discussions began when the shah's third wife, Empress Farah Diba, came to Mayo for a medical examination in 1978. Farah Diba was accompanied by Ardeshir Zahedi, the Iranian ambassador to the United States. Her attending physician invited the Iranian dignitaries to a formal dinner at Mayo Foundation House. Farah Diba helped to make this a special occasion by contributing large quantities of caviar brought in via her private plane. Adding to our enjoyment of the dinner, Zahedi presented each of us with a gift from Iran and later sent a note of praise for Mayo "on the extraordinarily high standard of care which you maintain." Not long afterward, political upheaval began in Iran. The Ayatollah Ruhollah Khomeini coordinated an upsurge of opposition, demanding the shah's abdication. With Reza Pahlevi's exile from Iran in 1979, the possibility of Mayo's involvement in Iran came to an end.

However, this did not put an end to the question of Mayo's expansion beyond Minnesota. Errett L. Cord, known for the sporty and technologically advanced automobile of the 1920s and 1930s that bore his name, first posed the question. (One famous Cord owner was architect Frank Lloyd Wright, who enjoyed driving the car from Taliesin, his home near Madison, Wisconsin, to Taliesin West in the Arizona desert. The Cord became a victim of the Great Depression. Cord sold the remnants of his auto business in 1937 and moved to Nevada, where he became a wealthy broadcaster, real estate developer, and state legislator.) After treatment at Mayo, Cord proposed giving a large sum to create a Mayo Clinic in Reno, where he had retired.

Mayo considered but courteously declined Cord's generous offer. Reluctant to accept the decision, Cord asked Emmerson Ward to come to Reno as a personal favor to evaluate the site. Ward, who was then chair of the board of governors, accepted the invitation and took with him Atherton Bean, chair of the board of trustees, and John R. Hodgson, chair of the board of governors' Extramural Practice Committee. Cord and his chauffeur met them upon arrival in Reno aboard Bean's private jet. Cord dismissed his chauffeur, saying he would drive the party to downtown Reno himself. With Ward sitting beside him in the front seat, Cord took off at considerable speed, commenting nonstop. He turned to the right and the rear as he spoke to make certain all three guests could hear him. Ward had to grab the steering wheel each time the car veered sharply and repeatedly to the right.

After two days in Reno meeting with the city's leading physicians and the dean of the developing medical school, my colleagues returned impressed by the quality of medical care available in Reno, but Mayo again declined Cord's invitation to develop a clinic there. Instead, the board suggested he fund a worthy cause at the Mayo Clinic in Rochester. This did not suit Cord, however. While disappointed he had not made a gift, the Mayo trio was relieved Cord did not drive them back to the airport! Later, I heard that when Cord mentioned the automobile tour of Reno to one of his lawyers, the response was, "Oh, so you've got your driving license back?"

Mayo Clinic Jacksonville

Though Mayo turned down some possibilities, it did decide in the long run to expand beyond Minnesota. Now there are three Mayo Clinics—the original one in Rochester, one in Jacksonville, Florida, and one in Scottsdale, Arizona. The Jacksonville clinic came about through the efforts of longtime Mayo patient James E. Davis, a founder of Winn-Dixie Stores, the largest supermarket chain in the southeastern United States.

A resident of Jacksonville, Davis became a contributor to the Mayo Foundation around 1948. In the mid-1970s, during a discussion with his physician about the cold Minnesota winters, Davis wondered whether Mayo might make its services available in the Sun Belt, where many older people lived. He proposed to arrange financial support for a Mayo Clinic branch near St. Luke's Hospital's proposed new facility. The oldest hospital in Florida, St. Luke's opened a $60 million facility in 1984 on a fifty-acre parcel of land donated by Davis, a trustee of the hospital since 1952. W. Eugene Mayberry, chair of Mayo's board of governors, told Davis that Mayo considered his offer an exciting opportunity.

Consequently, a group from the board, including internist Hugh Butt and me, flew to Jacksonville in October 1979. Davis took us on a helicopter tour of the area and later drove us to the proposed site. In his station wagon were three guns; he said he always carried them as a precaution. On the approach to the proposed site, which lay in an area he owned in the growing southeast quadrant of Jacksonville, we crossed a stream with a wooden bridge with the sign, "Chappaquiddick Bridge." We were able to guess his political views.

Davis left Butt and me to wander the property. Davis had let loose hordes of pigs; when he needed meat, he shot one. Also, the Jacksonville Transportation Authority had left four pits on the property after taking fill for J. Turner Butler Boulevard. The pits had filled with water, creating four lakes—inhabited by alligators. Butt, originally from Virginia, asked whether I had ever heard an alligator call. I had not. My colleague put his hands to his lips and made a strange noise. In a few moments several alligators slid from the water toward us. I learned later that Davis—who used the call to get the alligators' attention when he wanted to feed them—had taught it to Butt.

Butt recalled a meeting with Davis and W. Eugene Mayberry at which Davis offered to donate fifty acres if Mayo would build a clinic on the site. "J. E., that's not enough for a shithouse!" replied Butt in his direct way. Davis offered additional acres. Mayberry agreed to appoint a task force to assess the opportunity. Headed by Thane Cody of the board of governors, the task force recommended a "Mayo practice" outside of Rochester—at Jacksonville.

When word leaked out that Mayo might place a facility in Jacksonville, some members of the local medical community publicly opposed the idea, perhaps concerned that they might lose patients, Davis said. As a result, the board of governors rejected the task force's recommendation. Davis did not give up, however, and he repeated his enthusiastic proposal for a Mayo Clinic in Jacksonville when he came to Rochester again in March 1981. Mayo was still interested in the possibility of locating a clinic in Jacksonville, if it could resolve the opposition. As a result, James and Flo Davis donated 141 acres to Mayo in December 1982 but did not publicize the gift. Mayo was required in the deed to build a clinic within five years or the property would revert to St. Luke's Hospital or the Greater Jacksonville Community Foundation Donor Directed Fund.

Many of us at Mayo shared a concern that the federal government might create a national health care plan tying payment to whether patients obtained care in their own states. This would be a disaster for the Mayo Clinic in Rochester, since its patients come from all over the country and all over the world. Many thought Mayo should consider establishing centers elsewhere in the country as a precaution. The board of governors therefore decided to proceed with the opportunity in Jacksonville.

Jacksonville was ideal for its location in the Southeast, a rapidly growing region. Its high quality of life includes recreational opportunities and a thriving business community. Mayo also recognized that many senior citizens in the Midwest regularly spend part of each winter in Florida and that clinic physicians could see them there.

Although Jacksonville had few large multispecialty group practices and no medical school, Mayo was concerned that local physicians might see the new clinic as a threat to their own medical practice and so arranged to talk with them. At the same time, we were concerned with licensing Mayo physicians in Florida, where strict laws prevent visiting doctors from practicing medicine while on vacation there. Davis and his colleagues lobbied Florida's governor and key politicians, and the state legislature passed an act allowing Mayo doctors to practice in Florida. It limited practice to the Mayo Clinic and the number of physicians to thirty-five. This custom legislation encouraged Mayo but also worried local physicians who moved to exclude Mayo doctors from the staff of St. Luke's Hospital. Gradually, we convinced them that we were colleagues, not competitors. (Today, Mayo doctors recruited to the clinic in Jacksonville become licensed in Florida in regular fashion.)

The reasons for establishing the clinic were compelling. Licensure questions were resolved, the opposition was subsiding, and the land was donated. With all in order, the board of trustees voted in 1984 to establish a Mayo group practice in Florida. But the decision's delay precluded the opportunity to build the new clinic adjacent to St. Luke's Hospital. Instead the clinic is about seven miles away.

The first building on the Mayo Clinic's 140-acre site in Jacksonville honors James and Flo Davis and the entire Davis family. The primary architect of the building was Ellerbe Associates of Minneapolis, while Hammel, Green, and Abrahamson of Minneapolis created the interior. The Reverend Billy Graham gave the invocation at the dedication of the Davis Building on October 3, 1986, and speakers included Mayor Jake Godbold of Jacksonville, Mayo CEO W. Eugene Mayberry of Rochester, and Mayo Clinic Jacksonville CEO Thane Cody, an otologic surgeon at Mayo since 1963. The clinic opened ten days later.

Before construction of the new clinic, Davis held a luncheon at his club in Jacksonville and invited his business colleagues, many of whom had personal obligations to him. During the lunch, the host introduced those from Mayo and described to his colleagues the importance of Mayo's coming to Jacksonville. As they left the luncheon, he said, they would find a table with a letter for each of them stating their requested contributions. To our knowledge, all met his expectations! Sitting beside me at that lunch was the editor of the local newspaper, the *Times Union*. We learned we both had roots in County Donegal in northwest Ireland; indeed, we had grown up in small towns only three miles apart. Whether or not it was the result of our new friendship, Mayo got positive publicity in his newspaper.

The five-story facility, located fourteen miles from downtown Jacksonville, just three miles from the Atlantic Ocean, was staffed primarily by personnel from Mayo Rochester so that Mayo traditions would continue. On the initial staff were thirty-five Mayo-trained physicians in most medical and surgical specialties and 160 allied health staff. In its first year, there were 11,098 patient registrations from forty-seven states and seventeen foreign countries, and the initial staff increased to fifty-six physicians and 330 allied health staff. By its fifth year, Mayo Clinic Jacksonville had more than ninety thousand patient registrations and patients from all fifty states and seventy-five foreign countries. To meet the influx, Mayo Clinic Jacksonville completed a $30 million, eight-story expansion to the Davis Building in 1998. This and other expansions pushed the total investment to more than $300 million. By 2002, the clinic had 323 medical staff and 188 residents, fellows, and students in training.

The inpatient facilities of Mayo Clinic Jacksonville are in St. Luke's Hospital. Because St. Luke's existed before affiliating with Mayo in 1987, it was committed to community physicians who admitted patients to the hospital. St. Luke's primary purpose now is to support the practice of Mayo physicians, although the hospital continues its open staff policy. In addition, Florida's regulatory environment has favored maintaining the two institutions separately. As a result of these and other factors, Mayo Clinic Jacksonville and St. Luke's maintain their own governing boards but have some common members. The hospital board represents both Mayo and community physicians. In 2003 St. Luke's Hospital celebrated 130 years of service to Jacksonville. While the merger has been mutually beneficial, Mayo has long-range plans to build a new teaching hospital for tertiary medical care closer to the clinic. These plans are contingent upon the sale of St. Luke's, as well as obtaining additional financial support from benefactors.

In Jacksonville, the Davis School of Medical Sciences supports programs in medical education and research. Telecommunication between the

Jacksonville and Rochester facilities enhances patient care and permits shared educational programs. The Birdsall Medical Research Building at Mayo Clinic Jacksonville was dedicated in 1994. Completed in 2001 is the Griffin Cancer Research Building, the first building on the Jacksonville campus devoted exclusively to cancer research. It is named for longtime Mayo patients and benefactors C. V. and Elsie R. Griffin.

Mayo Clinic Scottsdale

In 1984, the same year the board of trustees voted to establish the clinic in Jacksonville, the trustees also voted to establish a third Mayo group practice in Scottsdale, Arizona. Mayo chose Scottsdale for its location on the eastern side of the rapidly growing Phoenix area, the heart of growth potential in the Southwest. Mayo purchased 139 acres of land in northern Scottsdale—bordered by mountains on the north and west—and the clinic opened in 1987. Because the five-story stucco facility harmonizes with its surroundings, two floors of the 164,000-square-foot building are below grade to preserve the mountain views. The exterior of the building is reminiscent of Mayo's home state, incorporating veined pink stone quarried in Minnesota with gray-green slate from England, the birthplace of William Worrall Mayo. The $45 million building has 112 examining rooms, a radiation treatment center, a pharmacy, and a 188-seat auditorium.

Richard W. Hill of the Mayo Rochester staff became CEO of the Scottsdale clinic, initially staffed with thirty Mayo-trained physicians and a paramedical support staff of eighty to 120, most from Arizona. When Mayo Clinic Scottsdale opened, the medical staff mainly used Scottsdale Memorial Hospital North, only five minutes away, for inpatient care and service. Mayo sought a merger with the hospital, but when the hospital rejected it Mayo announced plans in 1996 to construct its own hospital. The clinic purchased a 210-acre plot in northwestern Phoenix and opened the hospital in 1998.

The medical CEO chairs the boards of governors of the Mayo Clinics in Jacksonville and Scottsdale. And—as at Rochester—the majority of members come from the medical staff. The three boards report to the Mayo Foundation board of trustees to ensure maintenance of the Mayo principles in each organization. Under the governance of the Mayo board of trustees, the same triad of medical practice, education, and research applies in Jacksonville and Scottsdale as in Rochester, as well as the same principles of salaries, benefits, and administration.

high blood pressure

In 1979, near the end of my service on the board of governors, I proposed that Mayo establish a division to enhance the care provided to patients with hypertension. My interest in high blood pressure came largely from my research and involvement with the American Heart Association, which had formed the Council for High Blood Pressure Research in 1949 to encourage increased research on hypertension. The council publishes *Hypertension,* a journal devoted to research on the disease. I also had served as a member of the National Heart, Lung, and Blood Institute's Hypertension Task Force in 1976.

Irvine Page of the Cleveland Clinic, a doyen of research about disease, recognized the complexity of events that cause a chronic increase in arterial blood pressure. Optimal care of a patient with hypertension thus requires several specialties to work together, including experts in the kidney, the endocrine system, and the arterial blood vessels. From its inception, the Mayo Division of Hypertension organized around multispecialty cooperation. Established in 1982, the division includes knowledgeable clinicians and clinical (as well as basic) investigators. Recognizing the mosaic of abnormalities involved in hypertension, the new division added researchers in clinical pharmacology to advise on the optimal drug therapy for the individual patient.

Cameron Strong became the first head of the new division. He had trained with Jacques Genest, the scientific director of the Clinical Institute of the University of Montreal and an acknowledged expert in high blood pressure, and David Bohr at the University of Michigan, internationally known for basic studies on complex factors that regulate blood vessels. When Strong came to Mayo, he taught me and my colleagues how to conduct research on isolated blood vessels.

vascular medicine

The Division of Hypertension brought many advantages to Mayo's patients. Given my forty-year-long research on blood vessels, I was interested in Mayo's consideration of a center for vascular disease. Throughout my research, I had sought the complex mechanisms regulating blood vessels in health and the changes in vessels caused by disease. As president of the American Heart Association, I became convinced that diseases of blood vessels cause as many deaths in the United States as accidents, cancer, infections, and all other diseases. Blood vessel diseases include atherosclerosis, diabetes, high blood pressure, high cholesterol, and obesity. Together, they affect more than one in four Americans.

Despite the scale of the problem, attracting strong candidates to train as medical specialists in the vascular diseases, either as full-time clinicians or as clinician-investigators, has become increasingly difficult in recent years in the United States. One reason is the absence of subspecialty boards in these diseases. In large medical institutions, many disciplines contribute to the care management of patients with vascular disease. The involvement of internists and subspecialists in cardiology, endocrinology, hematology, rheumatology, neurology, radiology, neurosurgery, and cardiovascular and vascular surgery may result in fragmented care.

In 1989, nine years after my service on the board of governors, I chaired a committee looking into how Mayo could improve its care of patients with vascular disease. The Steering Committee on Vascular Medicine and Biology had twelve members representing groups involved with vascular disease. Early in 1991 we reported that advances in practice, education, and research would dictate consideration of the vascular system as a single system with diseases affecting the total system—this, rather than the traditional view of the system as separate anatomic divisions. The committee also declared that advances in the understanding, treatment, and prevention of vascular disease would depend increasingly on the close interaction of clinicians, clinician-investigators, and basic scientists. Training programs providing an understanding of the normal and abnormal functions of the total vascular system would be important too.

As a consequence of our report, the board of governors formed the Vascular Center Organizing Committee, which claimed fifteen thousand square feet in the Eisenberg Building of Rochester Methodist Hospital. The single location was optimal for the diagnosis and treatment of patients with vascular disease, including medical, neurological, and surgical consultations. The space also included laboratories for noninvasive cerebral and peripheral vascular testing. In addition, the space would be a learning resource center for educational programs in vascular medicine for medical students, residents, and those undergoing specialty training in vascular medicine. Mayo established fellowships in vascular disease, including training in research for those planning careers in clinical practice. Even though graduates may not continue their research, their experience at the Vascular Center teaches them the value of original thinking and initiative.

Major funding for the Gonda Vascular Center—the first of its kind in the world—came from the Leslie and Susan Gonda Foundation of Los Angeles. Named in their honor, it was dedicated in 1992. Between 1993 and 1996, the total number of patients treated at the Gonda Vascular Center for diseases of the arterial vessels, as well as for venous and lymphatic diseases, increased from a little more than ten thousand to almost twenty-one thousand per year.

The Gonda Vascular Center will triple in size to forty-five thousand square feet when it moves onto the fourth floor of the new Gonda Building on the Mayo campus in Rochester. Built with funds from an additional financial contribution to Mayo by the Gonda Foundation, the Gonda Building integrates the activities of each of the vascular medical specialties to enhance patient care. This not only provides a comprehensive approach to the clinical diagnostic and laboratory evaluation of patients with vascular disease, it also achieves an overall integration of clinical, education, and research activities in vascular disease throughout Mayo.

In 1992, the year of the dedication of the Gonda Vascular Center, I chaired a task force on vascular medicine for the American Heart Association. All the relevant disciplines were represented, and the task force report complemented the opinions expressed earlier by the Mayo committee I chaired. It recommended that medical institutes consider integrating practice, education, and research in a vascular center. We reasoned that coordinating educational programs and integrating vascular biology with clinical vascular medicine would translate advances in vascular biology into diagnostic and therapeutic interventions. Viewing the vascular system as a single system would permit clinicians, clinician-investigators, and basic researchers to cooperate in advancing vascular biology and medicine and enhancing the diagnosis, prevention, and treatment of vascular disease.

Things began to move after the AHA approved the report of the task force in 1993. It was time to recognize—despite the technical advances, including drug therapy, of the past twenty years in diagnosis and treatment—that the fundamental causes of vascular diseases remained hidden in the complexity of cellular events. The National Institutes of Health had already recognized the importance of gaining new knowledge to enhance the prevention and cure of vascular disease by establishing the U.S. Vascular Disease Academic Awards in 1992. Awardees serve as the focal points for interdisciplinary interactions in vascular medicine and enhance clinical, educational, and research programs. In April 2000, five major professional groups—the American College of Cardiology, the Society of Cardiovascular and Interventional Radiology, the Society for Vascular Medicine and Biology, the Society for Vascular Surgery of the United States, and the International Society for Cardiovascular Surgery—jointly sponsored a national conference, "Vascular Centers 2000: Best Practices in Interdisciplinary Collaboration."

Mayo held its first Mayo Vascular Symposium in 1996, and included a John T. Shepherd Lecture, which my friend and former research fellow Paul M. Vanhoutte delivered. The second Mayo Vascular Symposium, "Advances and Controversies in the Multidisciplinary Management of Vascular Disease," took place in Rochester in September 2000. Peter Gloviczki, an outstanding Mayo vascular surgeon from Budapest, chaired the symposium, jointly sponsored by Mayo, the American Venous Forum, and the International Union of Angiology. John C. Burnett Jr., a distinguished investigator of the cardiovascular system and director for research at Mayo, gave the second Shepherd Lecture—"Novel Strategies in the Prevention of Atherosclerosis." One session was "The Multidisciplinary Management of Vascular Disease: The Role of the Vascular Centers." In his introduction, Gloviczki recognized my role in the creation of the Gonda Vascular Center at Mayo. Presentations following his remarks showed the progress in developing other such centers in the United States, including the University of California's Gonda Vascular Center in Los Angeles, the Multidisciplinary Management of Vascular Patients at Stanford University in Palo Alto, California, and the University of Rochester (New York) Vascular Center. Thom W. Rooke, chair of the Gonda Vascular Center, described Mayo's progress in the final presentation.

The solutions to vascular disease lie in genetic dysfunctions, as emphasized at the 1996 symposium, "Research Initiatives in Vascular Disease: Vascular Gene Transfer: Models of Disease and Therapy," sponsored by the National Heart, Blood, and Lung Institute of the NIH, the International Society for Cardiovascular Surgery, and the U.S. Society of Vascular Surgery. With the mapping of the human genome now complete and many genetic studies in animals under way, the treatment of vascular disease in humans likely will be among the first applications of emerging gene therapy. This will require the close interaction of all concerned with vascular diseases—molecular biologists, clinician-investigators, and clinicians.

The necessity of continuing to train physician-scientists (clinical investigators) becomes ever more clear. Such specialists understand both the clinical problems and the increasing knowledge of genetic mechanisms. They must decide when it is appropriate to go from bench to bedside. The National Heart, Lung, and Blood Institute's decision in 2000 to fund "Programs of Excellence in Gene Therapy for Vascular Diseases"—five centers for five years at $3 million per center per year—demonstrates the importance of gene therapy. I am proud that Mayo was the trailblazer.

The United States is not alone in the advance against vascular diseases. Cardiovascular mortality represents around 40 percent of all causes of mortality before the age of seventy-four years in nearly every European country. The nineteenth World Congress of the International Union of Angiology recognized the importance of vascular centers in May 2000. Held in Ghent, Belgium, the congress was organized by one of my former fellows, Denis Clement, then chair of the Department of Cardiology and Angiology and dean of the medical school in Ghent. Clement convened the evening session, "Milestones in Vascular Medicine," and asked me to be its opening speaker on "From Basic Science to Clinical Medicine: Views on the Past, Present, and Future." He invited several important nonmedical Belgians, including Queen Fabiola, to attend the session. He emphasized the importance of explaining in ordinary language the new era in the application of genomics to the prevention and cure of vascular disease and urged me to stress that geneticists, clinician-investigators, and clinicians in vascular disease must come together to do so.

All of my work as a member of Mayo's board of governors dovetailed well with my concurrent term as a Mayo Foundation trustee, a position I held for twelve years between 1969 and 1981. Not only would I have the opportunity to join visionaries in directing the future of the clinic, I would come to know my fellow trustees as some of the most extraordinary movers and shakers of the twentieth century.

6

serving as a Mayo trustee

When my term ended in 1980 on the Mayo Clinic board of governors, I was still very much involved with Mayo Foundation's board of trustees, which I had joined in 1969 when I became the clinic's director for research.

Rather than involve itself in routine operations, the board of trustees remains a sounding board for major directions the Mayo Clinic wishes to take, such as the establishment of its development program, the Mayo Medical School, and the Practice Integration Project that resulted in the addition of the Jacksonville and Scottsdale clinics to Mayo's medical practice. The trustees are advisers and counselors who have ultimate financial responsibility for the Mayo institution. That includes resource allocation to salaries and benefits and to supplies and services, as well as allocation to capital expenditures and support for programs in education and research.

The Mayo Foundation board of trustees includes internal trustees from the staff and external trustees from a diverse array of other institutions. From government the board has welcomed senators, future Supreme Court justices, and a former vice president and president. From corporate America the board has included the heads of General Motors, Johnson Wax, Honeywell, and International Multifoods. Banking, communications, publishing, education, science, industry – all and more have been well represented on the board.

More than "a private trust for public purposes" – as described by former trustee and Supreme Court justice Warren Burger – the Mayo Foundation board represents the consummation of the ideals of the Mayo brothers: that is, a vision of the highest quality patient care through the integration of practice, education, and research.

Mayo Foundation board of trustees

The Mayo Foundation began in 1918 when William and Charles Mayo dedicated Mayo's assets and earnings in perpetuity to medical education and research rather than to the benefit of any individual. The Mayo brothers believed that no one should receive so much money that his or her children would not need to work. The Mayos wanted what they had built to outlive them as a public benefit. Their decision was in accord with the transfer in 1915 of a substantial portion of their personal fortunes to the University of Minnesota to begin the Mayo Graduate School of Medicine.

On October 8, 1919, the Mayo brothers established the Mayo Properties Association by conveying ownership of Mayo Clinic's property and assets to the new nonprofit association "in the faith that the Clinic and its operation and its privilege and opportunities to serve mankind may survive the donors." Later they changed the name to Mayo Association, then to Mayo Foundation.

By creating the nonprofit association and initially endowing it with the lion's share of their personal wealth, Dr. Will and Dr. Charlie dissolved the original partnership "and put all members on salary," thus ending the large sums of money the partners had earned up until that time (as evidenced by their large homes). Thus, Will Mayo turned over his home—now Mayo Foundation House—to the staff in 1938 as a place where men and women of medicine could exchange ideas for the good of mankind. It fulfills that purpose to this day. Only one of the clinic's original partners—Christopher Graham, a brother of Edith Graham Mayo, Dr. Charlie's wife—resigned as a consequence of the decision to create a nonprofit association. A veterinarian before he became a physician, Graham turned to breeding Holstein cattle until his death in 1952.

Each staff member at Mayo is salaried, and anyone starting at the bottom of the scale reaches the peak after five years. Hence, even relatively new staff members have the same income as senior members of the same specialty. To determine appropriate stipends, the Mayo Foundation board of trustees and others refer to annual national analyses of the salaries of specific medical and scientific disciplines. After they reach the salary cap, Mayo's medical and scientific staffs depend on cost-of-living increases. Mayo's salary system does not depend on the number of patients a staff physician sees or on the number of surgical operations he or she performs. Neither is there a profit-sharing system. No Mayo patient need worry that a matter of self-profit will affect the quality of care.

At Mayo, no one has tenure. Chairs of departments serve no more than ten years, sufficient time to plan and implement appropriate changes. In many medical centers, such appointment ends only at retirement, without consideration of the chair's continued ability to lead. Younger members in such a system consequently have no opportunity to assume leadership. A department chair at Mayo receives a modest salary increase (which continues after he or she steps down). Because of this long-established procedure, everyone knows that a changeover has nothing to do with someone's leadership qualities. Before appointing a new chair of a department, the board of governors' Personnel Committee seeks the opinion of every member of the group through interviews. The board of governors makes the final decision, based upon the committee's recommendations.

The Personnel Committee ensures the quality and performance of Mayo's professional staff. It determines, for instance, whether staff members are performing satisfactorily and researches the cause of any problem. If the committee decides that a problem is primarily social in nature (such as difficulties in personal relationships), the staff member has every opportunity to rectify the matter. During my service on the Personnel Committee, I persuaded my colleagues that, for problems related to professional competence, Mayo allow the staff member to take sabbatical leave to increase his or her professional competence within a specified time at another appropriate institution.

The policy of compensation through annual salary has been important to the evolution of the coordinated group practice of medicine that is Mayo. Under terms established by the Mayo brothers, the clinic leased facilities from the Mayo Foundation. At first the annual rent was the amount remaining after payment of the clinic expenses, which included an annual bonus for staff. Changes in the tax code dictated that the foundation review this arrangement just at the time I joined the board in 1969. To meet the IRS rules for tax-exempt status, Mayo discontinued the bonus system and reorganized under one legal entity, the Mayo Foundation.

All activities formerly divided between the clinic and foundation now fell under the foundation through three arms, or divisions. The clinic and its system of committees, responsible to its board of governors, remained as that segment of the unified institution conducting medical and surgical practice. The Research Administrative Committee retained its responsibility to supervise all programs of research and clinical investigation. The new Division of Education would conduct the Mayo Graduate School of Medicine, the Mayo School of Health Sciences, and ultimately the Mayo Medical School. Under the 1969 reorganization, the Mayo Clinic board of governors retained its function as the executive committee of the Mayo Foundation, responsible for overseeing Mayo's continuing programs and for setting broad institutional policy, using institution resources appropriately, and making long-range financial plans. The board of governors also has the power to act on behalf of the Mayo Foundation board of trustees between quarterly meetings.

The Mayo Foundation board of trustees grew in 1969 to include all the members of the board of governors and the public trustees. The board of trustees selects its chair, vice chairs, and other officials from its membership without regard to class of membership. The maximum size of the Mayo Foundation board of trustees is thirty, with up to sixteen positions reserved for public trustees, a majority of the board.

The public trustees' primary purpose is to protect the interests of those who receive care at the Mayo Clinic. They also bring the value of their expertise to Mayo. A public trustee, for example, chairs the Investment Policy Advisory Committee, which has primary fiduciary responsibility for Mayo's investments. The committee establishes an overall strategy to be carried out by professional portfolio managers. The committee chair is a prominent and respected national figure; past chairs have included two former chairs of the Federal Reserve Board, the editor of an international financial journal, and the head of a major trust company.

I interacted with Mayo's board of trustees between 1966 and 1987 in a variety of roles—as director for research and director for education, as a member of the board of governors, as an internal trustee, and as a member and chair of the board of development. During my twelve years on the Mayo Foundation board of trustees, as well as during my service to Mayo's board of development, I worked with a remarkable group of public trustees, many of whom I profile here. From corporate America, the government, the sciences, and points in between, they brought to the board their wisdom and vision in shaping Mayo's future. None were perhaps more visionary than the board chairs I served under: International Multifoods' Atherton Bean, Honeywell's Stephen F. Keating and Edson W. Spencer, S. C. Johnson and Son's Samuel C. Johnson, and Tennessee's Senator Howard H. Baker Jr.

Atherton Bean

Atherton Bean, chair and CEO of International Multifoods Corporation, joined the Mayo Foundation board of trustees in 1964 and served twelve years. His election as chair in 1969—the fiftieth anniversary of the foundation—marked the first time a public trustee had held that position. Bean's grandfather, Francis Atherton Bean, established the New Prague

Flouring Mill in 1892 in that Czech immigrant community in Minnesota. Flourishing under its Robin Hood Flour brand, New Prague Flouring Mill became International Milling Company in 1910 and International Multifoods in 1970, one of the largest food companies in the world.

Atherton Bean graduated summa cum laude in chemistry from Carleton College in Northfield, Minnesota. He went to business school at Harvard, then to Oxford as a Rhodes Scholar, where he earned a master's in economics, philosophy, and politics. He joined his family's business in 1937 and became its CEO after World War II, when he worked with the Office of Price Administration and with U.S. Army Intelligence.

In addition to his work as a Mayo public trustee, Bean's other public service included chairing the Carleton College board of trustees, the Ninth Federal Reserve Bank District, and the Minneapolis Society of Fine Arts. He had a great sense of humor: each time he came to Mayo for medical advice from the staff, he joked that he always left with a piece of him missing! He was also generous. Whenever one or more of us on the board went on a fund-raising journey on behalf of the Mayo Foundation to another part of the United States, he made available his private plane, greatly facilitating our endeavors.

Bean laid the foundation for employing the experience and skill of talented external trustees in guiding the Mayo Foundation, understanding the broad issues, and not getting sidetracked in the minutiae of the day-to-day. He defined his responsibilities at Mayo as the opportunity to provide a layman's view of the medical world and to draw upon his executive experience to counsel upon professional-related problems of a wider nature. He was aware of the outside forces operating upon medicine and of the problems unique to doctors. As an executive, he saw Mayo's three-part concept of patient care, education, and research as a practical prototype for future technical developments in medicine. He emphasized the importance of keeping the institution human and maintaining the principles of Mayo's founders, namely that patients should always know they are of paramount concern. Mayo may have endless committees, Bean once remarked, but it's also "a model for its effective management of a large concentration of confident, competent, highly-trained people who are continuously motivated toward the reach that exceeds the grasp."

Stephen F. Keating

Another outstanding business executive, Stephen F. Keating, former chair and CEO of Honeywell International, succeeded Atherton Bean as chair of the Mayo Foundation board of trustees in 1976. A diversified technology and manufacturing company, Honeywell serves customers with aerospace products, control technologies, automotive products, power generation systems, specialty chemicals, and electronics.

A worthy successor to Bean, Keating was first elected to the board in 1971. He gave invaluable assistance as we discussed academic disaffiliation from the University of Minnesota. When we discussed growth, Keating arranged for each internal trustee to meet individually with external members experienced in such matters. The external trustees advised that we had no choice but to grow, that we must be mindful of resultant challenges and maintain our principles—what we called "the spirit of Mayo."

Samuel C. Johnson

Samuel C. Johnson, CEO of S. C. Johnson and Son, succeeded Stephen Keating as chair in 1983. Johnson was the fourth generation of his family to head the Johnson Wax firm, founded in 1886 and headquartered in Racine, Wisconsin. The company manufactures products for household cleaning, insect control, personal care, and home storage.

Johnson, elected to the board in 1967, often entertained us with tales of his father, Herbert Johnson, and architect Frank Lloyd Wright, who designed both the S. C. Johnson and Son Building and the Johnson home in Racine. Samuel Johnson recalled what his father had said of Wright (whose difficult personality was legendary): "First we were working together, then he was working for me, then I was working for him." After Wright completed building the corporate headquarters and the family's house, Herbert Johnson discovered that both roofs leaked. Once, when he was hosting a dinner party at his home, it began to rain. When water dripped through the leaky roof onto the dining table, he telephoned Wright, who simply advised putting a bucket on the table to catch the water!

The Johnsons are longtime major benefactors of Mayo, having provided funds to construct the Samuel C. Johnson Medical Research Building at Mayo Clinic Scottsdale, which is engaged in determining the genetic basis of many diseases. On the topic of giving, Sam Johnson was fond of saying, "My father passed on to me a certain condition—I wouldn't really call it a 'disease'—of philanthropy. It's the one condition Mayo Clinic has never tried to cure!"

"A great company needs a great spirit," he also said. "It's something that transcends the balance sheet. It's almost mystical." Reflecting the opinion of the Mayo brothers, he believed that the Mayo Clinic embodies that spirit. When he retired from the board of trustees in 1990, Johnson had served twenty-three years—longer than any other public trustee.

Edson W. Spencer

Mayo tapped a second CEO of Honeywell, Edson W. Spencer, to chair its board of trustees. Appointed a trustee in 1984, Spencer is a graduate of Williams College who spent two years as a Rhodes Scholar at Oxford University before joining Sears Roebuck in Venezuela, then Honeywell in 1954. After serving as Far East regional manager in Tokyo, he became Honeywell's corporate vice president for international operations in 1965 and executive vice president in 1969, when he also became a director of the company. Spencer became president and CEO of Honeywell in 1974 and four years later its chair.

Spencer, a native of Chicago, was also active as chair of the advisory council of the Humphrey Institute of Public Affairs at the University of Minnesota, a trustee of the Minneapolis Foundation, chair of the Ford Foundation, and a director of CBS and Boise Cascade. He was a member of the international advisory board of Bosch, A.G., a trustee of the Carnegie Endowment for International Peace, and a member of the Council on Foreign Relations.

"Health care constitutes the most compelling issue on the domestic agenda today," Spencer wrote in 1991. "The severity of this problem's impact on the American people and on our economy makes change inevitable. At Mayo, we believe that change must incorporate those aspects of the present system that have enabled American medicine to attain an unparalleled level of quality." Mayo's public trustees, he said, serve as a resource in making decisions that help the institution remain successful, medically as well as financially, lending prestige as ambassadors to the outside world.

Howard H. Baker Jr.

Senator Howard H. Baker Jr. of Tennessee succeeded Edson Spencer in 1996 as chair of the Mayo board of trustees and served for two years. Baker joined the board in 1985 on the recommendation of trustee Cyrus Vance. He won recognition in 1973 as vice chair of the Senate Watergate Committee investigating the administration of President Richard M. Nixon. Baker became Senate majority leader, then served as White House chief of staff under President Ronald Reagan. Before entering politics, he was an attorney and businessman in his hometown of Huntsville, then in Knoxville. Both his father and stepmother (Irene Bailey Baker) served in Congress. His father-in-law was Everett Dirksen of Illinois, the longtime Republican leader of the Senate. After the death of his first wife, Baker married former Senator Nancy L. Kassebaum of Kansas, the daughter of 1936 Republican presidential candidate Alfred M. Landon.

Baker admired Mayo's reputation. He saw similarities between members of the Mayo board of trustees and the Senate. "As I looked around the room," he said after his first board of trustees meeting, "I saw leaders of great authority and respect in the nation. As Senate majority leader . . . I presided over a group of thirteen committee chairmen, all with great influence and national reputations, all strong personalities. That was not always easy. Half of them were running for president, and the other half were thinking about it."

Current events shortened Baker's term as board chair. By the time his term started, the serious medical consequences of tobacco smoking had been amply demonstrated. Minnesota attorney general Hubert H. Humphrey III pressed a strong legal case against the tobacco industry, and after a four-month trial on smoking-related diseases and forty years of industry efforts to downplay health issues, Minnesota won a landmark $7.1 billion settlement on May 8, 1998. Five months after the Minnesota case was settled, the tobacco industry negotiated a settlement with forty-six other states. Baker's Tennessee law firm agreed to defend the tobacco industry in subsequent litigation. Baker had no choice but to resign as an external Mayo trustee.

"the Minnesota Twins"

Of the distinguished individuals who have served the Mayo Foundation, I especially enjoyed working with future Supreme Court justices Warren Burger and Harry Blackmun, known as "the Minnesota Twins" during their time together on the court.

Warren Earl Burger was on the U.S. Court of Appeals when he joined the Mayo Foundation board in 1959. A Minnesota native, he had been appointed to the federal appellate bench by President Dwight D. Eisenhower. On May 21, 1969, President Richard M. Nixon named Burger the fifteenth chief justice of the Supreme Court. During his seven years on the Mayo Foundation board of trustees, he was an important adviser to the Mayo development program. Burger saw the wisdom in having public members on the Mayo board, saying, "Mayo's great medical and scientific staff has windows to the outside medical world, but it also needs windows to the outside lay world." When I wrote in 1987 to thank him for all his help during my years as chair of the board of development, he replied on stationery imprinted "From the chambers of the Chief Justice Burger—Retired." Even in his retirement, however, he was chairing the bicentennial celebration of the U.S. Constitution and admitted to me, "I hope to follow your example and shake off some of the heavy burdens of the Bicentennial program in a year or so."

Harry A. Blackmun was raised in St. Paul, Minnesota, and worked for a private law firm in Minneapolis for nearly twenty years before becoming the first full-time resident counsel in 1950 to Mayo Clinic and Mayo Foundation. Blackmun was a founder of Rochester Methodist Hospital and the author of its original articles of incorporation. In 1959 he was appointed to the Eighth U.S. Circuit Court of Appeals by President Eisenhower, but continued to live in Rochester. In 1969, after Justice Abe Fortas resigned from the Supreme Court, President Nixon sought the advice of Chief Justice Burger, who proposed Blackmun, his longtime friend and fellow Minnesotan. Blackmun was appointed in 1970 and served until 1994. His name will be forever linked to the 1973 decision that bore his signature, *Roe v. Wade,* also supported by Chief Justice Burger. That famous case effectively legalized abortion in the United States. I enjoyed knowing Blackmun, and I remember his talent for wiggling his ears, which greatly amused schoolchildren. "Maybe I will be remembered for this," he used to say. When I was director for education and dean of the medical school Harry Blackmun gave the key address at the 1980 graduation ceremonies.

LBJ

Former president Lyndon Baines Johnson began a four-year term as an external trustee on February 21, 1969. By 1968, Johnson had announced he would not seek another term as president because of widespread opposition to the war in Vietnam. He petitioned to become a member of the Mayo board of trustees, which he said would be both an honor and an opportunity to continue raising the quality of health care and research for all Americans.

In addition to the social measures enacted by Congress as part of his "Great Society" agenda—including Medicare and Medicaid in 1965—Johnson could claim a major global contribution to medicine for the role he played in the eradication of smallpox. In 1965 he appointed Donald Henderson, formerly of the Centers for Disease Control and Prevention, to head the World Health Organization's new Smallpox Eradication Unit. Henderson directed the unit until 1977, just before the world's last reported case of smallpox.

A former president of the United States on the board of trustees, a man who had focused the immense power of his office on solving a worldwide health risk—on one hand, the prospect was dizzying. On the other, it was problematic. Mayo tradition called for external trustees to propose the one to join them after a member had completed his or her term. Since Johnson had volunteered himself as a member, we asked senior administrator Slade Schuster to telephone each of the public trustees and ask for advice. All but one external trustee agreed to invite Johnson to join the board. Might the one trustee change his mind? He acceded and a short time later, Schuster's phone rang. It was LBJ. "Have I been elected?" he inquired. "Yes, indeed, Mr. President," Schuster replied. "Welcome aboard!"

Adding a former president to the board meant we had to make room for the Secret Service, so whenever we met, two agents inspected the building and checked our credentials. Adding this particular former president also meant we had to reexamine Mayo Foundation's policy regarding the serving of alcohol. We all knew Johnson enjoyed a drink or two. We were just as mindful that Mayo Foundation House did not serve alcohol, in deference to Will Mayo, a teetotaler. (In his memoir, *Mayo: The Story of My Family and My Career,* Chuck Mayo recalled an occasion on which his parents had invited President Franklin D. Roosevelt to dine at Mayowood. Chuck watched his Uncle Will suffer politely while FDR put away five martinis before dinner.)

Since dinner on the evening before the formal meeting of the trustees took place at Foundation House, what should we do? We decided to have drinks before dinner at the adjacent Damon House, then proceed to the Foundation House. As it happened, rain that evening forced us to reach the Foundation House by a low and narrow underground passageway. I escorted the former president, both of us well over six feet tall, both nearly doubled over, to our destination. We repeated this performance on three subsequent occasions. After that, the board reached a Solomonic judgment: the Mayo Foundation House could serve alcohol provided no formal medical or scientific meeting immediately followed dinner.

After a formal introduction by Atherton Bean, Johnson proposed at his first board meeting that the modest yearly honorarium provided to external trustees be terminated. Warren Burger had proposed the honorarium during his service as a trustee, but the board passed LBJ's motion unanimously. (Mayo does offer to pay expenses connected with attending meetings, but only a few external trustees request reimbursement.) Johnson's motion may have been based on the experience of Justice Abe Fortas, a 1965 Johnson appointee to the Supreme Court, who resigned after *Life* magazine revealed he had accepted a

$20,000 fee from a charitable foundation reportedly controlled by the family of an indicted stock manipulator.

Without hesitation, Johnson then proposed that the Mayo Clinic and Foundation solve the problems of heart disease and cancer in the next five years. I wondered whether he had in mind President Kennedy's famous speech about landing a man on the moon when he said that. We tabled this motion, realizing that Johnson's challenge was vastly more difficult than space endeavors. The answers to the causes of these most complex diseases involve the new era of molecular biology and genetics that is even now, more than thirty years after Johnson's motion, just in its infancy.

While public trustees are not involved in Mayo's day-to-day operations, five of them chair the audit, officer succession, development advisory, investment policy advisory, and nominating committees. In 1969, the board established a sixth standing committee on compensation of medical and administrative trustees, with Lyndon Johnson, Atherton Bean, and Sam Johnson as its first members. Since then, this committee of three public trustees must approve any salary change for internal trustees.

public trustees of the 1970s

New public trustees in 1970 were Edward N. Cole, president and CEO of General Motors; William McChesney Martin, chair of the Federal Reserve Board; Gerard Piel, editor and publisher of *Scientific American;* and Hugh D. Galusha Jr., president of the Ninth District Federal Reserve Bank, headquartered in Minneapolis.

As head of the world's largest corporation, Edward Cole sometimes advised associates to "kick the hell out of the status quo." Someone once asked him at a trustee meeting whether GM planned to make smaller cars. No, he answered—Americans wouldn't buy them. How times have changed!

William McChesney Martin, who chaired the Federal Reserve from 1951 until 1970, was a strong contributor to the Mayo board during his nine years as a trustee. A 1928 graduate of Yale, Martin at age thirty-one became president of the New York Stock Exchange. He served as chair of the Federal Reserve during the administrations of five presidents—Truman, Eisenhower, Kennedy, Johnson, and Nixon. Like most presidents, Johnson stewed over a rise in interest rates and pleaded to Martin in 1965, "You wouldn't raise the interest rate while a fella was having his gallbladder out?" (In a famous photo, Johnson gleefully pulled up his shirt to show reporters his scar from his gallbladder surgery, performed at the Mayo Clinic that year.)

I recall one occasion when Martin joined board of governors chair Emmerson Ward and me in paying a visit to William L. McKnight in Florida. McKnight, then in his eighties, was a founder of 3M Corporation and we wanted to gain his support for Mayo education and research programs. We were hopeful until McKnight turned to Martin with a litany of woes—recession, inflation, and the Watergate scandal. "Well," Martin began, "things look pretty bad." That's as far as he got. McKnight interrupted him: "I knew it. At a time like this, I wouldn't make a commitment to my grandmother."

Citing the nineteenth-century British politician Benjamin Disraeli—"Individuals may form communities, but it is institutions alone that make a nation"—Martin once declared that Mayo was helping to build our nation, telling sponsors of the Mayo Foundation in 1972, "Here is an institution that always kept the patient—the individual—in focus. . . . Mayo represents the very finest in American life."

I enjoyed a long friendship with Bill Martin and with trustee Gerard Piel and his wife, Eleanor, a distinguished defense lawyer. Piel was science editor of *Life,* then assistant to the president of the Henry Kaiser Company and its affiliates before he organized in 1946 (with Dennis Flanagan and Donald H. Miller Jr.) the publishing enterprise that has carried *Scientific American,* America's oldest periodical, well into its second century.

Piel declared he was "deeply interested in medical care as an interface between science and society. The ethical questions involved in making science work for people are raised in their most acute and sharpened form in medicine. Here at Mayo . . . [is] a very different kind of medicine from that in the large city—different in kind, in patient population, in organization."

Piel, who was a member of the Health Research Council of the City of New York and chair of its Commission on Delivery of Personal Health Services, served the maximum of three four-year terms as a Mayo trustee. He viewed the impact of science on individuals with guarded optimism, promoting ethical consideration of patients in the practice of medicine.

Following our many discussions on health care in the United States, Piel sent me a copy of a 1932 report published by the University of Chicago Press, *Medical Care for the American People.* Piel believed the issues raised by the report and the conclusions reached had "important lessons for everyone trying to reach agreement on medicine in America for the twenty-first century." I agreed, and found myself hoping that everyone involved with the current debate about health care—politicians, medical societies, medical administrators, and physicians—would read this report, still relevant more than seventy years later.

"Management is entirely lay and relatively unconcerned with professional standards," the report reads, adding that "much of the medical service has been obtained from the lowest bidder, although sometimes it is paid for at the workmen's compensation rates. Finally, this plan, instead of obtaining the economies and professional advantages of group organization and group practice, actually adds to the cost through expensive selling procedures and payment of profits to owners."

Hugh D. Galusha Jr. was a partner in a Helena, Montana, CPA firm until 1965, when he became president of the Ninth District Federal Reserve Bank in Minneapolis. The trustees were barely beginning to get to know Galusha when he died while snowmobiling with fifteen other men in his native Montana on January 31, 1971. The group was making its way from Red Lodge to Cooke in a snowstorm by way of Beartooth Pass. Near the top of the eleven-thousand-foot pass, the snowmobiles began to malfunction, and Galusha died en route to cabins beyond the summit. The cause of his death has not been established with certainty, but it may have been due to the effects of high altitude on the respiratory and cardiovascular systems. (My colleague Autar Paintal, from the Patel Chest Institute at the University of Delhi, demonstrated in animals the presence of what he termed J-receptors, or juxtapulmonary capillary receptors, in the lungs. These can be activated if the lungs start filling with fluid at altitude and cause severe respiratory discomfort due to a constriction of the airways.)

Three new public trustees joined the Mayo board of trustees in 1973: Joan Ganz Cooney of public television's Children's Television Workshop and developer of *Sesame Street,* the most successful children's show in the history of television; George Dillon, CEO of Butler Manufacturing Company in Kansas City, the world's leading producer of pre-engineered metal buildings; and Newton N. Minow of the Chicago law firm of Sidley and Austin and former chair of the Federal Communications Commission. In 1961, Minow described television as "a vast wasteland"—an epithet repeated by so many critics that Minow feared it would appear on his tombstone.

Historian Hanna Holborn Gray, president of the University of Chicago, became a Mayo public trustee in 1974. She was reared in an eminent German academic and scientific family: Her paternal grandfather was the director of a Berlin research institute and a physical chemist. Her mother had a doctorate in classical philology. The family came to the United States in the early 1930s after her father, European historian Hajo Holborn, lost his academic posts during the rise of the Nazis. (In the United States, Holborn joined the faculty at Yale.) A scholar specializing in the Renaissance and Reformation, Hanna Gray joined the faculty at Harvard before she became dean of the College of Arts and Sciences at Northwestern University in 1972, provost at Yale University in 1974, and its acting president three years later. In 1978, at the University of Chicago, she became the first woman to head a major university in the United States.

To Gray, Mayo's greatest strengths lie in its diversity. She noted that Mayo is among the nation's "great centers that go beyond the particular institution, beyond the particular region, even beyond the particular functions which they may emphasize, to be national resources. . . . It is only through the presence of such great national resources—which are private in origin and which at the same time have an effect on all of us—that the diversity and the constant redefinition of quality, of service and purpose in education, can be accomplished."

Joining the board in 1975 was Thomas J. Watson Jr., son of the founder of IBM and its chair and CEO during the company's most explosive period of growth. *Fortune* magazine described him in 1987 as "the greatest capitalist who ever lived, if creating wealth for shareholders is the best measure of a businessman's success." When he retired in 1971, IBM's capitalization was $36 billion more than when he took over from his father fifteen years before.

A lifelong Democrat and a staunch advocate of mutually verifiable reductions in nuclear arms, Watson was President Jimmy Carter's ambassador to Moscow. In 1956, as IBM was deciding whether to establish plants outside Poughkeepsie, New York, Watson met for dinner with the father of a deceased member of Watson's former World War II flight crew. Why not Rochester, Minnesota, for the plants, suggested his dinner companion, a lifelong city resident. As a consequence, an outstanding IBM facility was built in the community!

The new IBM presence had a direct effect on Mayo Clinic. At that time, the clinic was open for patient care on Saturday mornings. The work week at IBM, however, ran Monday through Friday. As both institutions grew, we realized they were competing for the same employees—IBM for its workforce,

Mayo for its nonmedical staff. As a consequence, Mayo stopped opening on Saturday mornings.

Catherine B. Cleary became a Mayo public trustee in 1977. An attorney, she was the former president, CEO, and chair of First Wisconsin Trust Company and a member of the boards of five other major corporations (AT&T, General Motors, Kraft, Kohler, and Northwestern Mutual Life Insurance).

Joan D. Manley joined Mayo as a trustee in 1979. In 1975, she became group vice president of Time, Inc., the first woman to reach such a high executive post with the largest book publisher in the United States. Formerly chair and CEO of Time-Life Books, she was the eldest child of a Polish immigrant who built a multimillion-dollar construction business in California.

Goethe's observation that "you cannot understand history without having lived through history yourself" certainly applied to Mayo trustee Cyrus R. Vance, who joined the Mayo board of trustees in 1980. During the Johnson administration, Vance served as deputy defense secretary. As secretary of state during the Carter administration, he became embroiled in the decision as to whether the Shah of Iran, Mohammad Reza Pahlevi, would be allowed to enter the United States. The shah, who had fled Iran after a popular revolt in January 1979, was suffering from lymphoma and wished to receive medical treatment at New York Hospital. The Carter administration's decision to let him enter the United States angered supporters of the Ayatollah Khomeini, who had returned from exile to Iran to establish a new regime. Khomeini denounced the United States as the "Great Satan," and Iranian students stormed the American embassy. They held fifty-two Americans hostage. Vance, who opposed an attempt in 1980 to rescue the hostages, resigned after the mission failed. Iran released the hostages after 444 days in captivity on January 20, 1981, the day Ronald Reagan succeeded Jimmy Carter as president.

public trustees of the 1980s

Among the business leaders who served on Mayo's board of trustees during the 1980s was Rawleigh Warner Jr., a top oil executive who began his career at Continental Oil before moving to Mobil Overseas Oil. Warner became executive vice president of Mobil International Oil in 1960, then president in 1965, then chair and CEO from 1969 until 1986. He served on the board of trustees from 1980 to 1992.

John Willard Marriott Jr., chair and president of the Marriott Corporation, served from 1986 until 1998. His father, John Willard (Bill) Marriott, founded the hotel corporation that bears his name. The elder Marriott was a picturesque figure. He and a partner opened an A&W Root Beer stand in Washington on May 20, 1927—the same day Charles Lindbergh landed in Paris after flying nonstop across the Atlantic Ocean. Years later, the two men met for the first time, and Marriott said to Lindbergh: "You and I went into business the same day, but you got all the publicity!"

Whitney MacMillan, chair and CEO of Minnesota-based Cargill, became a Mayo trustee in 1984 and served until 1997. As the largest commodity dealer in the world, Cargill buys, processes, stores, transports, and sells agricultural and other bulk commodities throughout the world. "Whatever the world birth rate for a given year, that's the number of people we can potentially serve," Whitney MacMillan once said.

On one occasion MacMillan arranged for Garrison Keillor, creator of that mythical Minnesota town called Lake Wobegon, to address the Mayo staff after a dinner. I was asked to introduce Keillor—no mean task! I tried to get into the spirit of the occasion by being humorous, wondering aloud what might have happened had William Worrall Mayo ended up in Lake Wobegon instead of Rochester. Keillor noticed my Irish accent at once, assuring me the Scots-Irish Presbyterians would be homeless among the Norwegian Lutherans of Lake Wobegon!

Whitney and Elizabeth MacMillan established the Management Scholars program at Mayo Foundation in 1994, providing an endowment to fund advanced management educational opportunities for Mayo physicians with demonstrated organizational leadership potential. Since 1996, eighteen doctors on the Mayo staff have become MacMillan Scholars at schools such as the Kellogg School of Management at Northwestern University and the Wharton School of Finance at the University of Pennsylvania.

Walter F. Mondale and Medicare reform

Although his appointment occurred after my time on the Mayo Foundation board, my wife and I have enjoyed knowing former vice president Walter F. Mondale and his wife, Joan, who also has a distinguished record of public service in Minnesota. A lifelong Democrat, Walter Mondale was elected attorney general of Minnesota in 1960, then served in the Senate alongside his friend and mentor, Hubert H. Humphrey. Mondale, who was Jimmy Carter's vice president from 1977 until 1981, ran unsuccessfully as the Democratic presidential nominee against Ronald Reagan in 1984. He served Mayo as a trustee from 1989 until 1993, when President Bill Clinton named him ambassador to Japan. Upon his return to Minnesota, Mondale joined the Minneapolis law firm of Dorsey and Whitney and rejoined the board in 1997.

Mondale's diverse and distinguished background and lifetime of public service made him an ideal candidate for the Mayo board of trustees. His willingness to serve and his personal philosophy of leadership outlined in his 1975 book, *The Accountability of Power,* have made him a valued and respected member of this governing body.

Speaking to the Mayo staff in September 1999, Mondale focused on what medical organizations such as Mayo might do to preserve Medicare. Yes, the paperwork is appalling, there are funding inequities from state to state, and pharmaceutical coverage was not included in the original Medicare bill (which Mondale cosponsored in 1965). But with all of its faults, Medicare is the only entitlement-sourced funding to cover the costs of graduate medical education. Congressional cuts in Medicare spending represent not only a decrease in patient care reimbursements, Mondale said, but also cuts in medical education.

Mayo Foundation favors transforming Medicare to a model similar to the Federal Employees Health Benefits Plan. This plan includes a basic set of benefits, flexibility in benefit design, multiple choices of insurance providers and options, and a defined government contribution that can be augmented by the individual to pay for additional coverage. This model maximizes individual choice and minimizes government micromanagement of the health care system, yet still allows the government to provide support for hospitals serving rural and low-income populations, as well as for research and education.

My experiences with the boards of governors and trustees have reinforced my belief in the Mayo system of government, based on the principle that the staff—medical practitioners and researchers—are here to serve the patients who seek our services, without regard to other considerations. This demands the close interaction of everyone on the medical staff. It also demands that we remain abreast of medical developments.

Debate continues around the world on the best way to deliver medical care, and I don't know whether any other major world medical center has adopted the Mayo system in its entirety. Our extensive system of committees, as some have observed, does not generate the rapid decision-making that other centers with highly paid nonmedical executives boast. But because medical colleagues make organizational decisions, the Mayo system ensures that they are acceptable to the staff. Administrators at Mayo assist the medical staff in implementing those decisions. At the same time, Mayo's distinguished public trustees, without whose approval no major decision may be implemented, ensure that Mayo sticks to its mission.

clinic and hospitals merge

In 1986 the Mayo Clinic merged with its associated hospitals, Rochester Methodist and Saint Marys. Over many long years, the relationships among the three institutions had been cordial and productive, with word-of-mouth agreements and no legal documents. Still, a merger offered clear benefits to all three parties. In an era of rapidly increasing hospital costs, much could be gained by integrating the two hospitals to minimize overlap. The hospital medical staffs were already members of the Mayo Clinic, so this posed no major concern, but Saint Marys Hospital needed to assure the Vatican of the preservation of the Catholicity of the hospital.

When Rochester Methodist and Saint Marys Hospitals became part of the Mayo Foundation in 1986, a sponsorship agreement provided for a sixteen-member board. The sponsorship board—comprised of Franciscan Sisters and lay colleagues—emphasizes the patient as first priority. The work of the board fosters compassion, trust, mutual respect, and spiritual support for patients, their families, and members of the health care team.

Charter House

Finalizing the hospital merger meant addressing relations between Mayo Foundation and a Rochester retirement center, Charter House, a subsidiary of Rochester Methodist Hospital Health Services. Charter House opened in 1985 but by the end of that year had rented only about half of its apartments. With its revenue considerably less than projected, Charter House approached Mayo Foundation for financial help. Subsequent discussions by the Mayo Clinic board of governors and the Mayo Foundation board of trustees recognized the inherent value of Charter House. Many of its residents were Mayo patients, Rochester residents, and emeritus members of the Mayo staff. The Mayo Foundation extended up to $12 million to Charter House, which not only resolved the center's financial difficulties, it also allowed the merger of Mayo and Rochester Methodist Hospital to proceed. With 245 units, Charter House today has a long waiting list for admittance—and an addition of forty-five assisted-living units, a library, and several shops for residents.

Another benefit of the merger of the Mayo Clinic and the hospitals involved fund-raising. Instead of seeking financial support from private donors, often with overlapping appeals, the Mayo Clinic and Methodist and Saint Marys Hospitals evolved into a single enterprise. Fund-raising became the responsibility of Mayo Foundation's board of development, which I joined three years after its establishment in 1969. As I was about to find out, becoming chair of development would be the capstone in my administrative responsibilities at the Mayo Clinic.

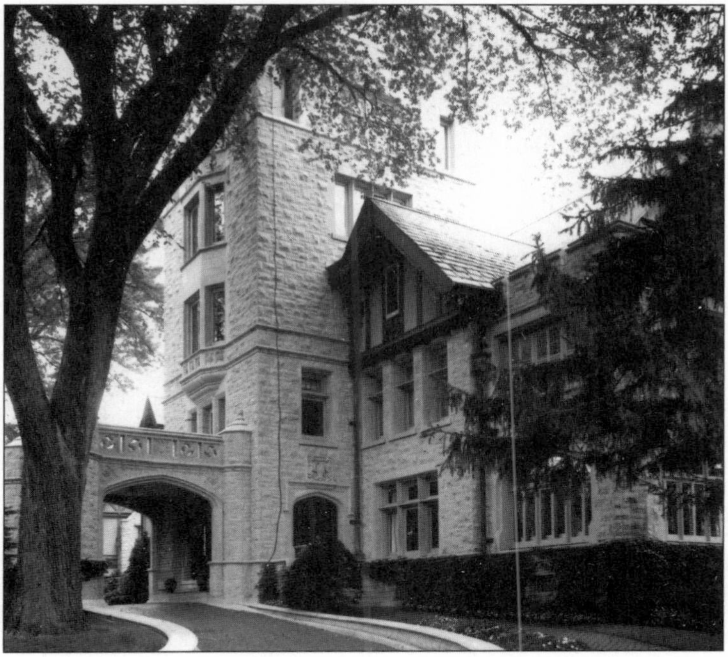

In 1938, the former home of William J. Mayo became Mayo Foundation House, a symbol of continuing medical education at the clinic and a reception center for visiting dignitaries. (MAYO PHOTO ARCHIVES)

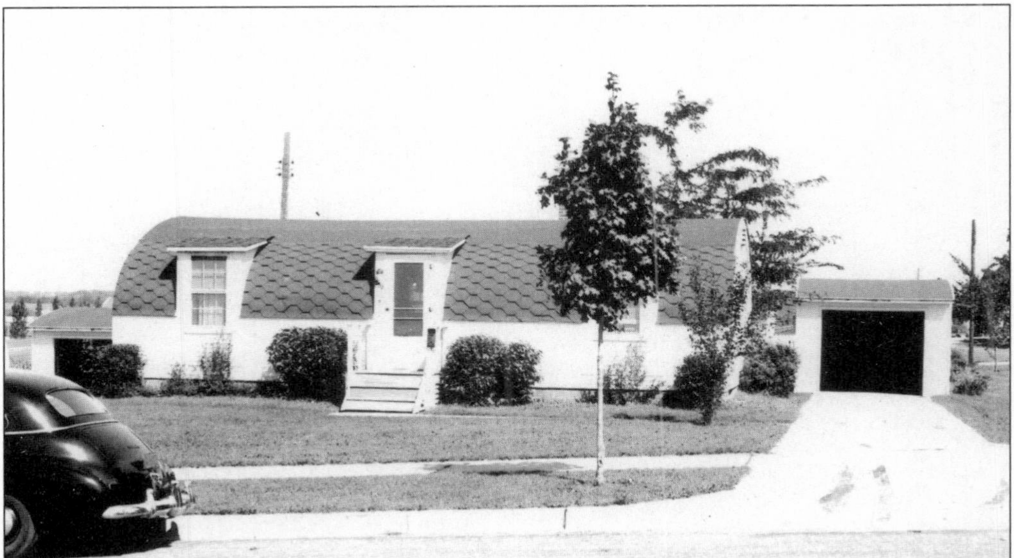

Post–World War II Mayo fellows lived in prefabricated Quonset houses. (MAYO PHOTO ARCHIVES)

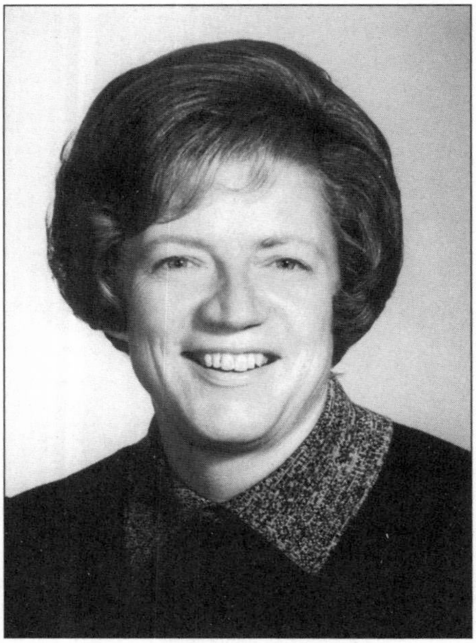

University of Chicago president Hanna Gray, a Mayo Foundation public trustee, addressed the Mayo Medical School graduating class of 1982.

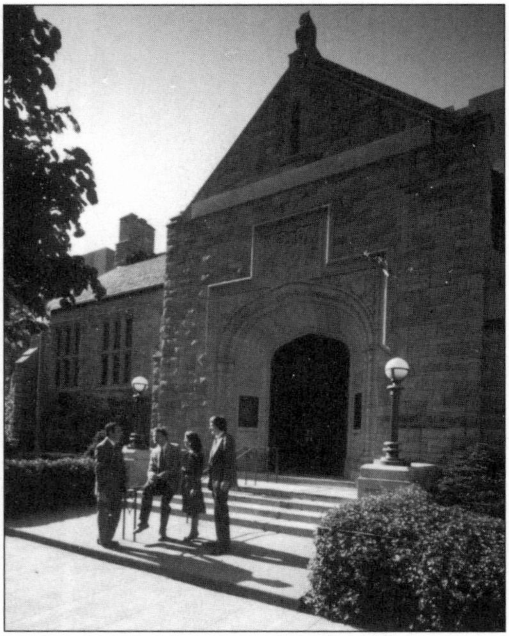

The Mayo Medical School in Rochester is the city's former public library. (MAYO PHOTO ARCHIVES)

The grounds of the Harwick Building and Harwick Plaza feature the sculpture *Four Square Walk-Through*, given by the Goulandris shipping family of Greece. The Mayo Building is on the left, the Plummer Building in the background. (MAYO PHOTO ARCHIVES)

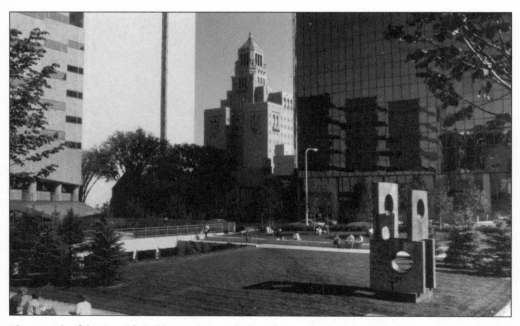

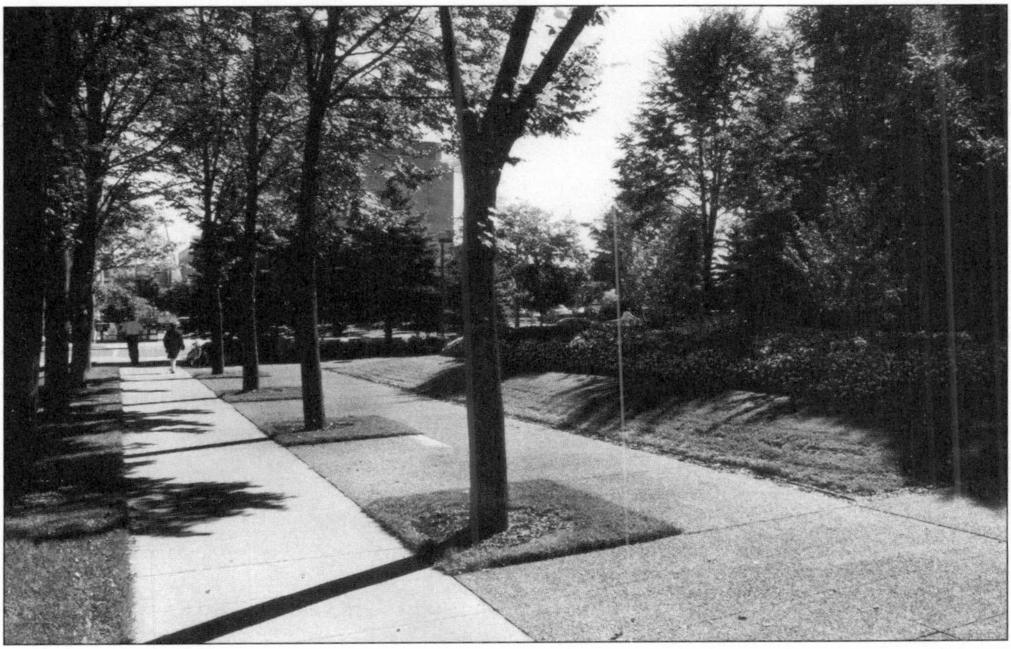

Abutting Harwick Plaza is a green space once occupied by a city street. (MAYO PHOTO ARCHIVES)

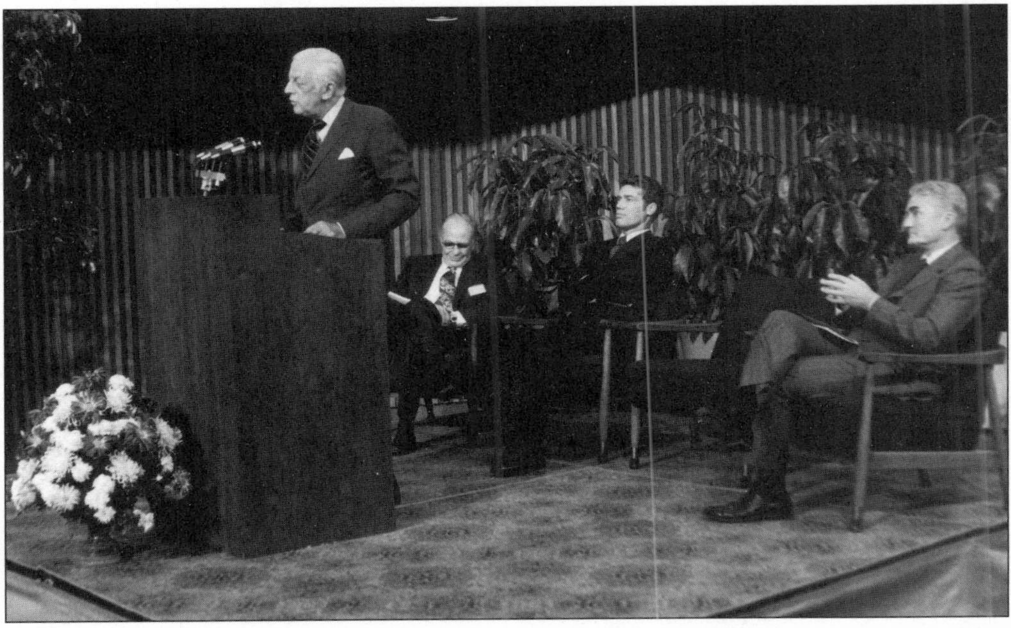

Actor Alistair Cooke speaks at the dedication of the Guggenheim and Hilton Buildings in 1974. Behind the speaker are (from left) Mayo board of trustees chair Atherton Bean, Minnesota governor Wendell L. Anderson, and Mayo board of governors chair Emmerson Ward. (MAYO PHOTO ARCHIVES)

***Man and Freedom*, a three-ton sculpture by Croatian-born Ivan Mestrovic, appears on the north facade of the Mayo Building in Rochester. (MAYO PHOTO ARCHIVES)**

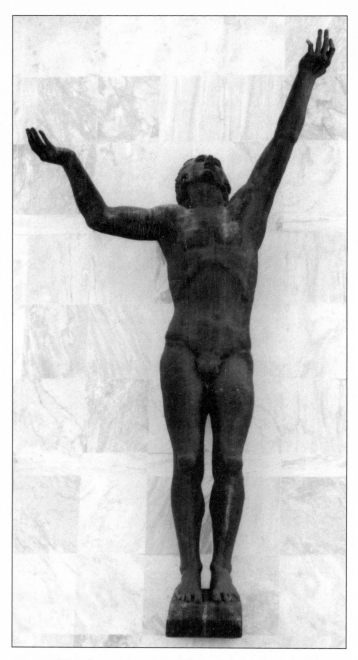

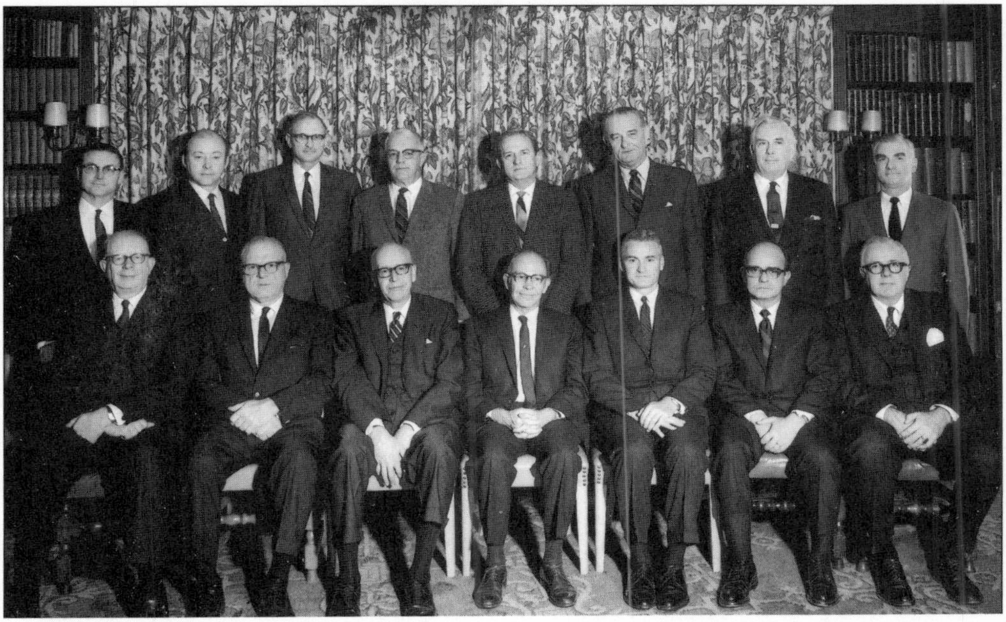

The Mayo Foundation board of trustees, February 1969. Standing, from left: Dr. Oliver Beahrs, Samuel C. Johnson, the author, Dr. William Sauer, Dr. James DuShane, Lyndon B. Johnson, Warren Burger, Robert Roesler. Seated, from left: Dr. Dwight Wilbur, Dr. J. Minott Stickney, G. S. Schuster, Atherton Bean (chair), Dr. Emmerson Ward, W. Clarke Wescoe, J. W. Harwick. (MAYO PHOTO ARCHIVES)

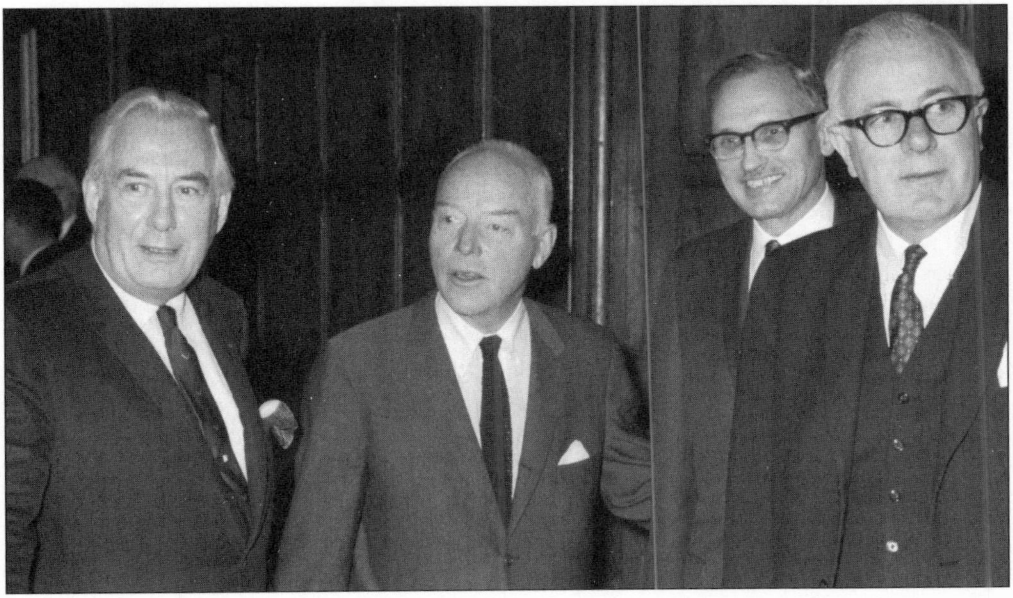

From left: Judge Warren Burger, Mayo surgeon James Priestly, the author, and Bill Harwick at a meeting of the Mayo Foundation board of trustees. (MAYO PHOTO ARCHIVES)

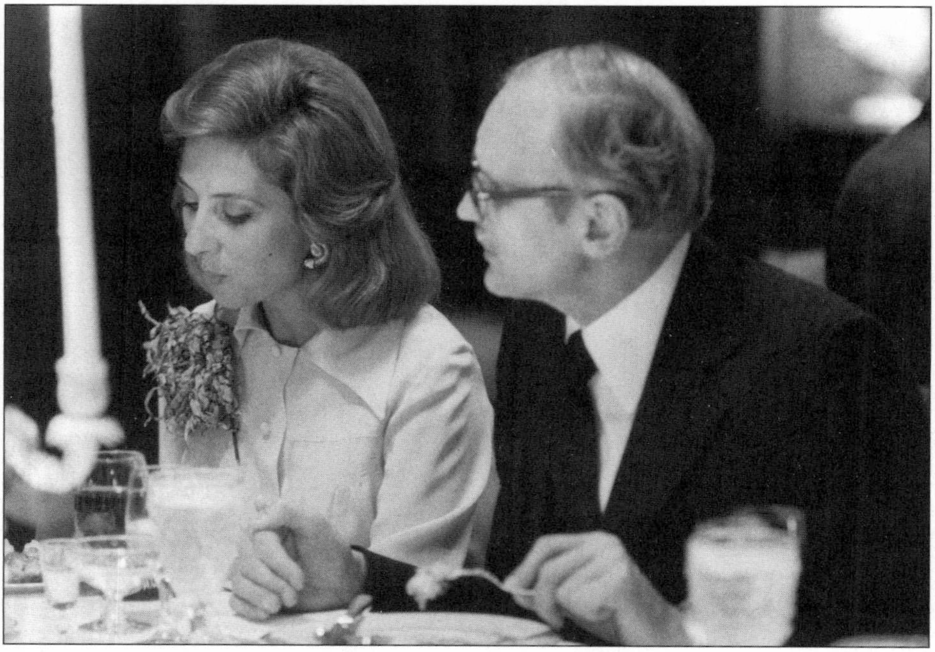

Farah Diba, third wife of the shah of Iran, and I attend a formal dinner at the Mayo Foundation House in early 1970. (MAYO PHOTO ARCHIVES)

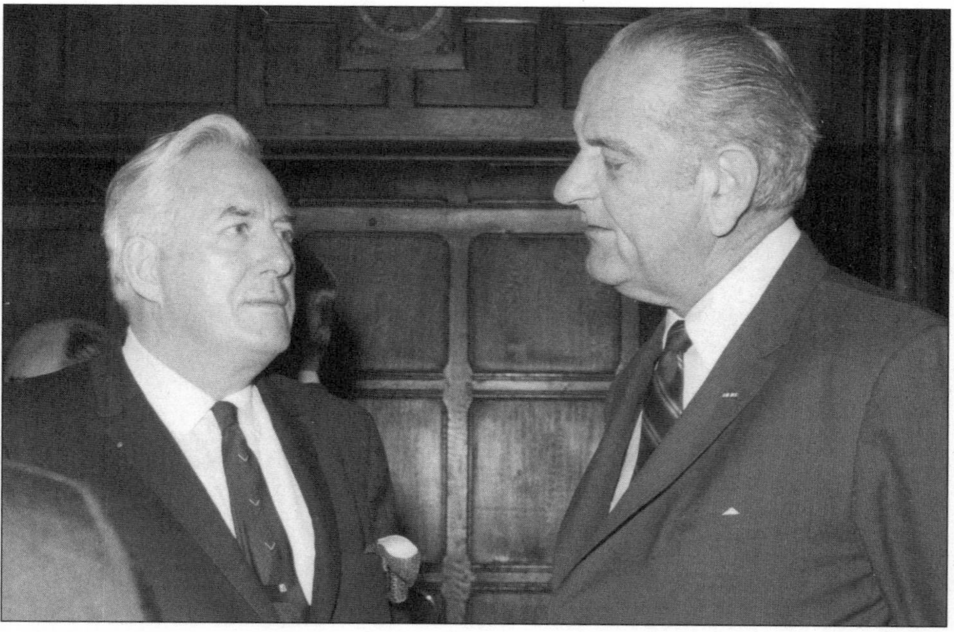

Judge Warren Burger (left) and former president Lyndon Johnson deliberate at a meeting of the Mayo Foundation board of trustees. (MAYO PHOTO ARCHIVES)

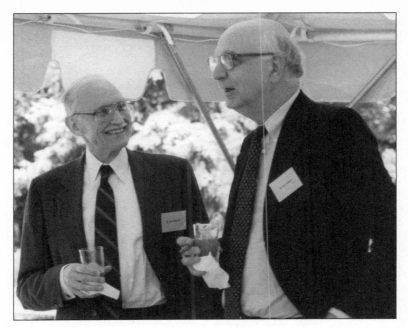

Paul Volker, Federal Reserve Board chair (right), and I chat in the garden of Mayo Foundation House at a trustees meeting. (MAYO PHOTO ARCHIVES)

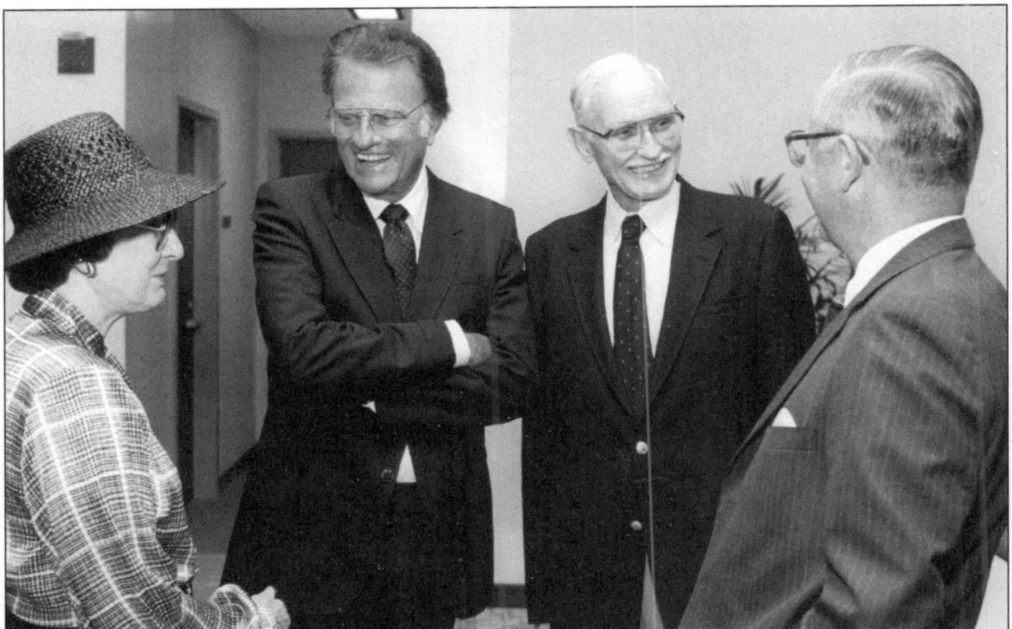

From left: Helen Shepherd, the Reverend Billy Graham, the author, and chief medical officer Thane Cody at the 1984 opening of Mayo Clinic Jacksonville. (MAYO PHOTO ARCHIVES)

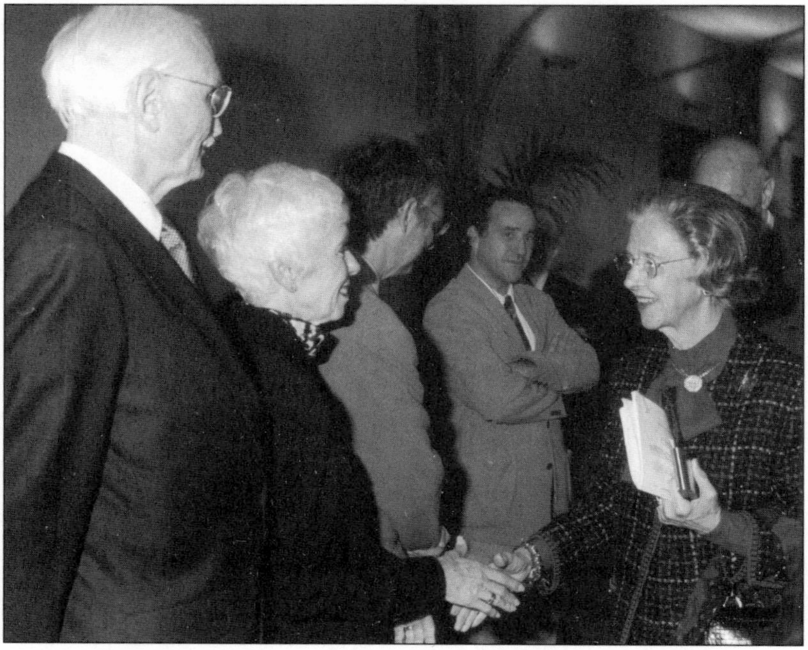

My second wife, Marion, and I meet Queen Fabiola of Belgium at the World Congress of the International Union of Angiology in Ghent, Belgium, in May 2000.

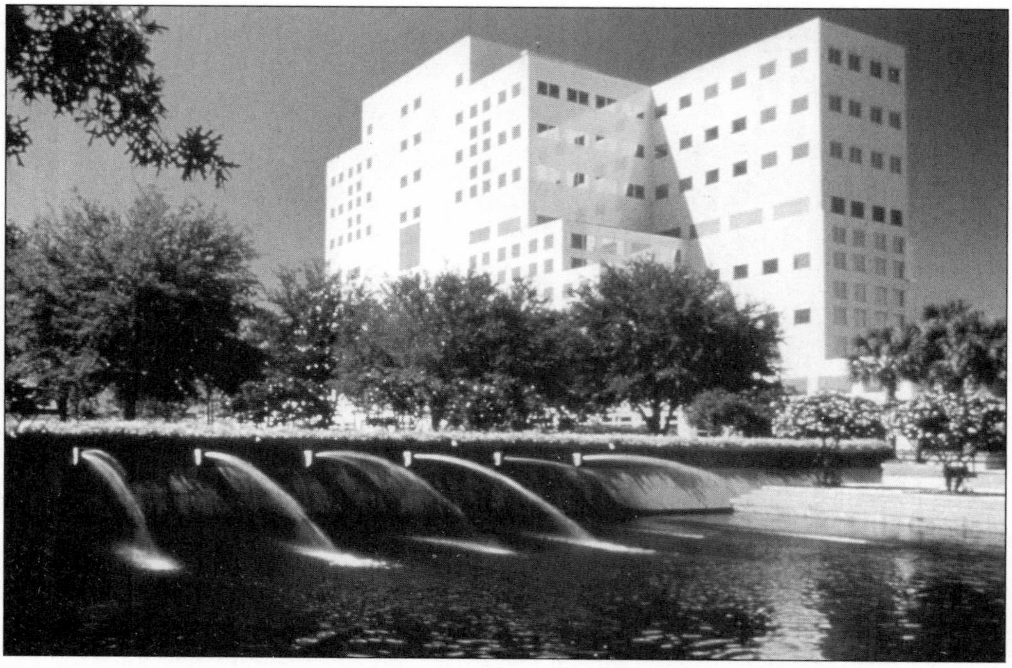

The Davis Building at Mayo Clinic Jacksonville. (MAYO PHOTO ARCHIVES)

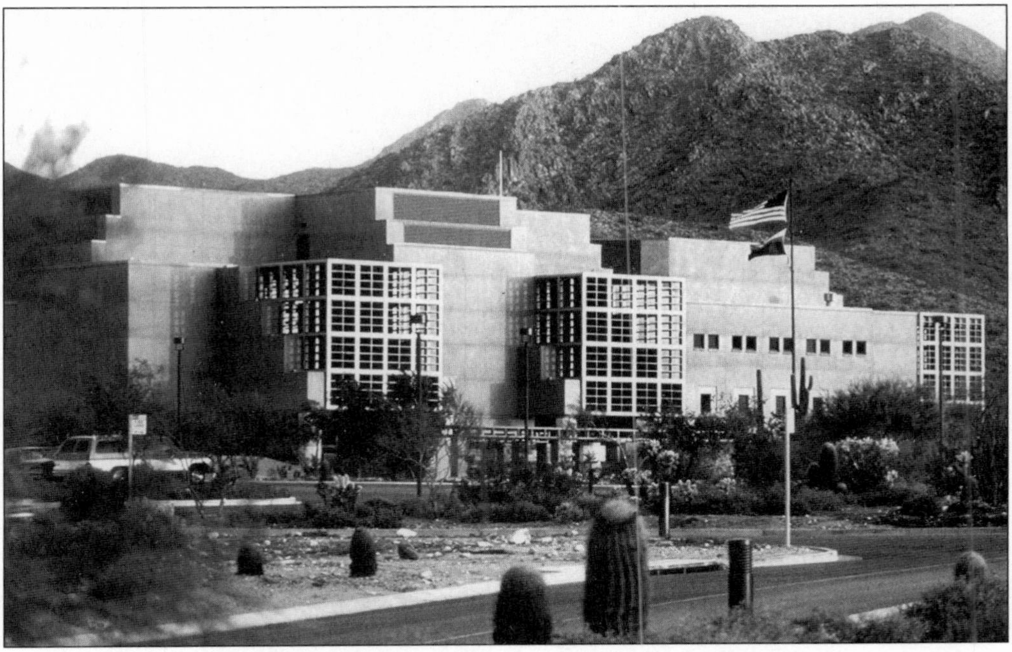

The design of the Mayo Clinic Scottsdale building harmonizes with its southwestern surroundings. (MAYO PHOTO ARCHIVES)

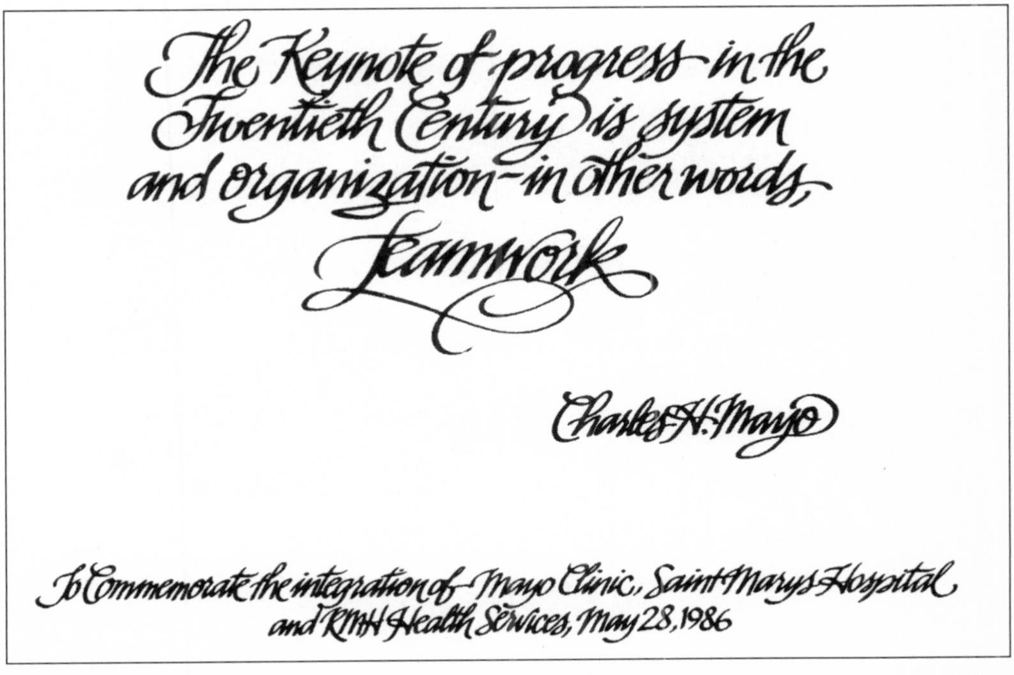

The Keynote of progress in the Twentieth Century is system and organization—in other words, Teamwork

Charles H. Mayo

To Commemorate the integration of Mayo Clinic, Saint Marys Hospital and RMH Health Services, May 28, 1986

Mayo commemorated its merger with Saint Marys and Rochester Methodist Hospitals in 1986 with an observation by Charles H. Mayo.

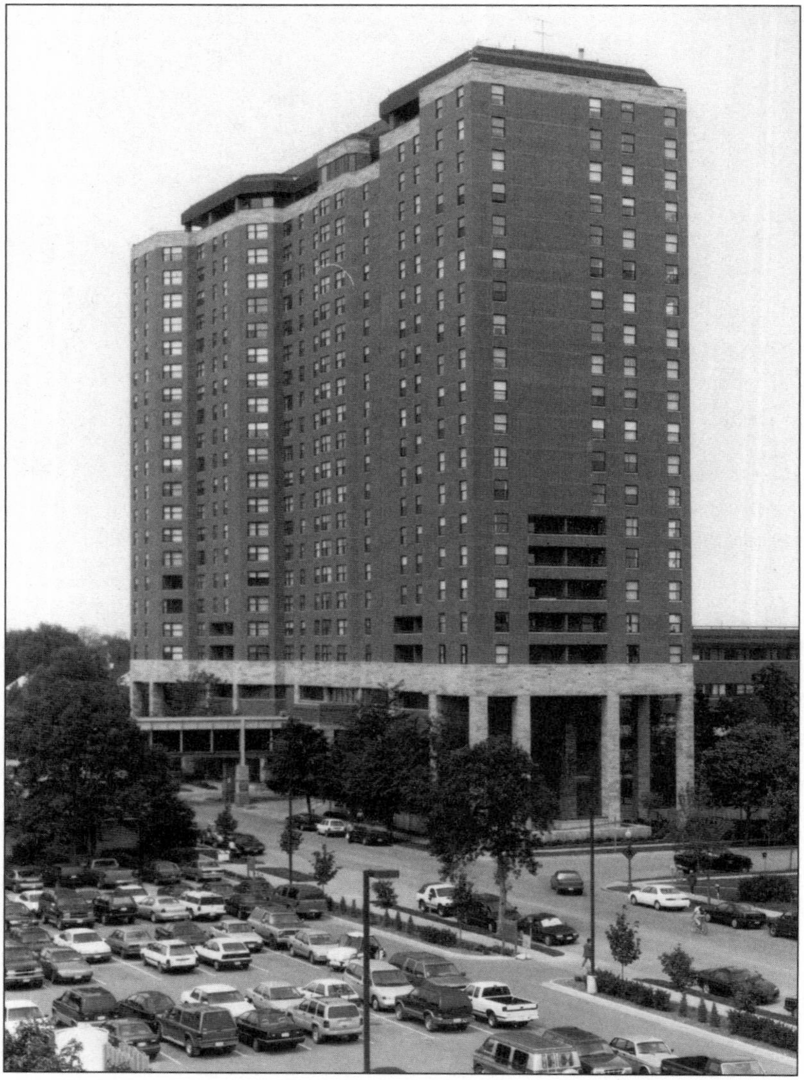

Charter House is linked to Rochester's subway and skyway system, making the retirement center accessible to the clinic and the downtown area through all kinds of weather. (MAYO PHOTO ARCHIVES)

7

fundraising for the future

The major impetus for establishing Mayo's development board was the trustees' challenge in 1969 to raise $33 million from non-Mayo sources before establishing the Mayo Medical School. More than three decades later, the development board continues to strengthen Mayo's education, research, and health care facilities programs through gifts from generous benefactors. The Gonda Building, the largest construction project in Mayo's history, for example, was funded by Leslie and Susan Gonda and integrates outpatient and inpatient services.

Contributions to the Mayo Foundation come from varied sources. Generous alumni give to the foundation via the Doctors Mayo Society, which was created in 1977. The foundation also administers bequests and other planned gifts made to the Mayo Legacy of Medicine, established in 1990. Many of those bequests, which have resulted in more than sixty endowed named professorships, came about through the efforts of Mayo's external trustees, whose reputations as national leaders act as an invaluable asset to all aspects of the Mayo enterprise, including the Jacksonville and Scottsdale clinics.

During my fifteen years on the board of development (from 1972 to 1987, the last four as chair), I had the great pleasure of meeting and working with major benefactors to Mayo, including Barbara Woodward Lips, who bequeathed $127.9 million to the Mayo Foundation – the largest single gift to the clinic. Charlton, Eisenberg, Siebens, Rappaport, Gonda – the names of these and several other benefactors grace many an atrium, hall, and building. Such generosity has ensured – and continues to inspire – Mayo's continuing legacy of medicine.

Mayo Foundation board of development

When Mayo Foundation established its board of development in 1969, an esteemed Mayo neurologist, Kendall Corbin, became chair. Shortly thereafter, Anthony S. Bridwell, director of development for Northwestern University, became its head administrator. Other members of the inaugural development board were Atherton Bean, chair of Mayo's board of trustees; Emmerson Ward, chair of Mayo's board of governors; Charles Code, director of Mayo medical education and research; Raymond Pruitt, director of the Mayo Graduate School of Medicine; endocrinologist Randall Sprague of the medical staff; Charles Owen, a medical research scientist; and two senior administrators, Slade Schuster and William Harwick.

Mayo's guidelines for its development program have been simple from the start: the clinic regularly seeks gifts to strengthen Mayo's education and research programs from those with good reason to support the Mayo effort. The board's first challenge was to raise $33 million, the amount Mayo's trustees had judged necessary to run the new Mayo Medical School for ten years. To begin, the board held "Industry Day at Mayo" in Rochester in 1970, its first organized presentation. A distinguished group of executives, representing some seventy major industries and large companies, came to see firsthand Mayo's innovative approach to the delivery of health care through group practice combined with education and research. Cohosts IBM and 3M announced leadership gifts, and the First National Bank of Rochester and Merck pharmaceutical company together pledged $1.2 million.

"This is the first time I've ever seen approximately a hundred of the nation's business leaders meet to inform themselves and attempt to make a contribution to the health of this country," said former president Lyndon Johnson, one of the three external members of the Mayo board of trustees who addressed the group. "Here, under the umbrella of a single institution, we have an opportunity to strike a blow against heart disease, against cancer and stroke, and against the shortage of medical personnel." In his typically colorful fashion, Johnson reminded his audience that American corporations were giving away only a fraction of the 5 percent of income they were allowed to give before taxes: "You people can give away a lot more to causes you believe in. Now why the hell ain't you doing it?"

After "Industry Day at Mayo," the Hill Family Foundation of St. Paul (now the Northwest Area Foundation) and the Bush Foundation of Minneapolis each committed grants of $1 million. A steady stream of corporate gifts from $100,000 to $250,000 came in from companies such as General Motors, Burlington Northern, Sears Roebuck, G. D. Searle, Andersen Windows, and

S. C. Johnson. Atherton Bean and several other public trustees, including William McChesney Martin and Samuel C. Johnson, also came through with commitments that, along with other gifts, amounted to around $4 million. By the summer of 1971, the board of development had about $16 million in hand.

Private gifts were not the only factor in our quest for start-up funding for the medical school. The ten-year projection of the state capitation of $8,000 per year for each student enrolled from Minnesota amounted to almost $11 million for the forty students enrolled each year. We could also count on an estimated $4 million from sources such as tuition, interest from gifts in hand, and a federal subsidy. As the mid-August reckoning with the board of trustees approached, the development board could count $31 million from all sources. The final $2 million came from commitments of alumni, several individual pledges, and a handful of late-blooming corporate gifts. A $450,000 grant from the Commonwealth Fund finally put us over the top. The board of trustees unanimously approved opening the Mayo Medical School in September 1972.

When I joined the board of development that year, it expanded and organized itself into working committees. The executive committee consisted of the chair of the board of development, the chair of the board of governors, the dean of the medical school, the director for research (me), the chair of administration, and the head of the Section of Development. The gift recognition committee established guidelines for the comprehensive program of donor recognition, while the staff development committee—composed almost exclusively of physicians—informed Mayo colleagues about the purposes of the development program and the need for their assistance.

Since development was new at Mayo, doctors naturally were reluctant to ask patients for gifts, even though patients are assured that the quality of their medical care is not related in any way to giving. As the doctors began to understand the low-key nature of our conversations with prospective givers, however, they became increasingly cooperative about the role they could play in raising funds for Mayo. The staff development committee contributes in numerous ways to increased advocacy by the medical staff. For example, it developed *For Tomorrow's Medicine,* a brochure outlining Mayo's history and goals that it distributed to some sixty thousand patients and other prospective donors. Today, the booklet *Friends of Mayo* is available throughout the Mayo campus, including Jacksonville and Scottsdale, and by mail to our many benefactors.

the Doctors Mayo Society

The Mayo Alumni Association launched the Doctors Mayo Society in 1977 to recognize the importance of philanthropic support to Mayo's threefold mission in medical practice, education, and research. Mayo alumni, senior administrators, trustees, and spouses are eligible for membership in the society, which includes more than two thousand individuals in fifty states and fourteen countries. The society's philanthropic support to date exceeds $31 million. Alumni raised $500,000 to fund the Mayo Alumni Center, located in the Siebens Building. This is important information for other benefactors, who sometimes ask what alumni do to provide funds.

endowed professorships

By 2003 Mayo had sixty-six endowed named professorships, which give donors the opportunity to honor someone such as a parent or spouse and which enable Mayo to honor a distinguished member of the staff. Mayo originally set the amount required for a named professorship at $1 million but in 1993 increased the amount to $2 million. Funds for such professorships go into endowment, and an institutional committee allocates income from the investment to a purpose consistent with the donor's wishes. The income from a professorship endowment is a component of standard institutional support, not a supplement; thus, the salary of the individual occupying a named professorship is paid through regular administrative channels.

The board of development informs the development policy committee of donations for established named professorships. The committee then appoints an ad hoc group to recommend candidates for the professorship based on his or her activities involving clinical practice, education, and research. The Mayo Foundation education committee reviews the recommendations. Aside from exceptional circumstances, the candidate for such a professorship must be a Mayo consultant with the rank of professor in the Mayo Medical School or must have been recommended for promotion to professor by the academic appointments and promotions committee. (I became eligible for a named professorship with my appointment as professor of physiology in the Mayo Graduate School of Medicine in 1962, and from 1977 until 1983 I was the Northwest Area Foundation Professor of Medical Education.) After approval, the Mayo Foundation board of trustees confers any named professorships. An individual may hold a named professorship as an active member of the Mayo staff but not beyond retirement. He or she continues to have all the rights, privileges, and obligations of a staff member of Mayo Clinic and Foundation.

George M. Eisenberg endowed several named professorships at Mayo, as have several of our external trustees, including Atherton and Winifred Bean, Alice Sheets Marriott, Whitney and Betty MacMillan (who also established the Management Scholars Program in 1994), and Thomas J. Watson Jr. The Whitney and Betty MacMillan Professorship in Ophthalmology honors Robert R. Waller, former chair of Mayo's Department of Ophthalmology and later Mayo's CEO. The Watson professorship honors Robert L. Frye, a Mayo cardiologist who served as chair of the Department of Internal Medicine and as president of the American College of Cardiology.

Mayo Legacy of Medicine

The inaugural meeting of the Mayo Legacy of Medicine, an organization of donors who have made generous bequests or other planned gifts to Mayo Foundation, took place in October 1990 at the Harold W. Siebens Education Building. Joining me as speakers were my successor as chair of the board of development, W. Eugene Mayberry; Mayo chief executive officer Robert Waller; board of governors chair emeritus Emmerson Ward; Mayo trustee and Hormel chief executive officer Richard Knowlton; Mayo emeritus administrator Robert Roesler; and National Planned Giving Institute director Robert Sharpe Sr. Together, we stressed that the standards set by Will and Charlie Mayo for medicine, social responsibility, and philanthropy would indeed continue in the spirit of "the Mayo legacy."

experiences with major benefactors

Many of Mayo's benefactors are longtime patients. The basis of their willingness to provide funds to help advance Mayo's principles is the relationship they enjoy with their Mayo physicians. Whenever a patient indicates an interest in making a gift, the physician refers him or her to the chair of the board of development. This practice dissociates the wishes of the patient from the particular interests of the physician and from the care of the patient. Board members also call on prospective donors who are earmarked by the Mayo Foundation development policy committee, the director for development, and the Department of Development, who coordinate the optimal approach.

As a member and subsequent chair of the board of development between 1972 and 1987, I was privileged to know a number of extraordinary benefactors. Together with my colleagues, we blended the donors' desire to give with the institution's needs.

Ruth Charlton Mitchell Masson

Ruth Charlton Mitchell Masson was the daughter of Earle Perry Charlton, a cofounder of F. W. Woolworth. Ruth's husband, Frederick M. Mitchell, owned a wholesale leather business in Philadelphia. Like her father, she directed much of her philanthropy toward the advancement of medicine, particularly by supporting cancer research and medical education. She and her husband supported the Charlton Memorial Hospital in Fall River, Massachusetts. After Mitchell died in 1960, she married Mayo surgeon James C. Masson in 1965. He died in 1975.

Ruth Masson provided funding to develop study facilities for Mayo medical students in what once was the Rochester Library. The Tudor Gothic building, designed by Rochester architect Harold H. Crawford, was constructed in 1936 and 1937 for $178,000. When the small library could no longer accommodate its clients' increasing demands, Mayo Foundation bought the building for $375,000 to make it the center of the new medical school's activities when classes first began in 1972. After Mayo made major improvements in 1985, it renamed the building the Ruth and Frederick Mitchell Student Center. The reading area of the former public library became Charlton Hall, a study and library, in honor of the donor's father.

Mayo honored Ruth Masson at the dedication of the student center on November 22, 1985, not only for the center itself, but also for the James C. Masson Professorship in Surgery, the Frederick M. Mitchell Scholarship Fund, and the Guggenheim Building's Charlton Hall, in honor of her father. She gave generously to the Ida S. Charlton Trust and the Earle P. Charlton Jr. Trust, honoring her mother and brother. "In addition to the services this building will render to medical education," I remarked at the dedication of the student center, "you have established the Ruth and Frederick Mitchell Research Trust for the securement of new knowledge of cancer and other diseases that afflict mankind. . . . All of us are the beneficiaries of your great generosity to Mayo."

A diagnostic and treatment facility, the Charlton Building was built with funds from a charitable trust estate by Ruth Masson. The initial six-story building was a 200,000-square-foot addition to the Mayo Clinic, adjoining Rochester Methodist Hospital. In November 1988, radiation oncology, transfusion service, venipuncture, pain clinic, anesthesiology offices, diagnostic radiology, nuclear medicine, and the obstetrics service moved into the building, dedicated in 1989 on the donor's ninety-eighth birthday. Mayo later added five floors to the Charlton Building during construction of the Gonda Building.

Ruth Masson died in February 1995 at her home in Rochester, at the age of 104. She once had told us she had one ambition in the last months of her life: to live longer than her earlier acquaintance, Rose Fitzgerald Kennedy. She achieved her wish by some days.

George Eisenberg

George Eisenberg's parents fled to the United States from czarist Russia at the turn of the century. They settled in Chicago, but when George was two, his father died, leaving his mother penniless to raise seven children. At age eight, George began selling newspapers in the city's Maxwell Street ghetto. (Other well-known Americans from the now famous neighborhood include CBS president William S. Paley, actor Paul Muni, and band leader Benny Goodman, as well as Admiral Hyman G. Rickover, father of the nuclear submarine, and Jack Ruby, slayer of Lee Harvey Oswald.)

When he was just twenty-one, George Eisenberg started the American Decal and Manufacturing Company in Chicago. He made a fortune by making decals for all occasions, including decals of the bald eagle for the U.S. Postal Service—one for every mailbox in the country. After the job was complete, the postal authorities realized they had made a mistake: they had wanted the eagles to face the same direction from both sides of the mailbox. They placed a second order for the same number of decals, all facing the opposite direction from the first. Thus Eisenberg realized an unexpected financial boost!

Eisenberg came to Mayo in the early 1950s, and, grateful for his care, he made generous donations to the clinic. Eisenberg was no stranger to philanthropy. Based on the experiences of his own family, he had been underwriting programs for the needy since 1934; by the time I first met him, he was supporting some thirty-five charities. In honor of his philanthropy to the clinic, Mayo named the George Eisenberg Building for him. I presided at the dedication of a sculpture of Eisenberg on May 9, 1983, inside the Eisenberg Building at Rochester Methodist Hospital. He specifically chose sculptor Avard T. Fairbanks of Salt Lake City, famous for his sculptures of Lincoln.

Eisenberg called his Mayo friends his extended family, and even kept a plaque on his desk that read "There's no fun like work"—a quote from Dr. Charles H. Mayo that Eisenberg had printed at his company and gave freely to his friends. He named the clinic the beneficiary of half his estate and established several professorships, including many in honor of his family: the Rose M. and Morris Eisenberg Professorship for his parents; the David Eisenberg, Michael M. Eisenberg, and Reuben R. Eisenberg Professorships for his brothers; and the Bernard Pollack Professorship for his nephew and forty-five-year American Decal employee. George Eisenberg also established the Charles H. Weinman Professorship in 1988 to honor American Decal's chief chemist, who was a Holocaust survivor.

George M. Eisenberg died in 1989, less than a week before his ninetieth birthday. Mayo had lost a great benefactor, and many of us a dear friend. Yet his philanthropic work lives on. Mayo Foundation received a five-year, $5 million research grant from the George M. Eisenberg Foundation for Charities of Chicago in 1998. This gift, which supports development of translational research and molecular medicine, is the largest single grant by the Eisenberg Foundation to any foundation or charity.

Harold W. Siebens

Harold Walter Siebens also was a longtime Mayo patient. Born in Storm Lake, Iowa, he grew up in St. Louis, where his father, Walter, began the American Sporting Goods Company. The elder Siebens later developed an amateur radio set with a signal so reliable and powerful that the navy asked him to help back up communication with an early expedition to the North Pole.

Harold Siebens was a keen sportsman, and when his father died in 1940 he took over the family business and made American Sporting Goods one of the top three suppliers of sporting goods in the United States. He sold the business in 1948 and set off with his family to fish and hunt in Alaska. As they drove through Alberta, Siebens said he "smelled oil." He acquired thousands of acres of land in Alberta for one U.S. dollar per acre. When oil was discovered a decade later, he resold his mineral rights to developers. As I recall, Dome Petroleum paid him upwards of $300 million.

To avoid paying U.S. taxes, Siebens settled in Lyford Cay in the Bahamas. He invited New York financier John Templeton to join him. Templeton moved his main office to Fort Lauderdale, Florida, and resettled in the British-owned Bahamas, where his investments flourished. (Templeton, who later became a British citizen and was knighted by Queen Elizabeth, established the Templeton Prize for progress in religion in 1972 to redress the fact that there is no Nobel Prize for religion.) Both Siebens and Templeton were concerned with the limited health care facilities in the Bahamas; any illness of consequence meant that they and other wealthy citizens had to fly to Miami. They asked me to see whether Mayo would consider establishing a clinic in Nassau, but my colleagues and I decided there were too many uncertainties for us to attempt this, despite an offer of financial assistance.

Technological advances make such a concept far more plausible today. At the request of the United Arab Emirates' ministry of health, Mayo recently developed a highly sophisticated telemedicine system that allows it to offer specialty medical resources and expertise to patients at Al Mafraq Hospital in Abu Dhabi. In consultation with colleagues, Mayo doctors review medical records and offer opinions on whether appointments at the clinic would be helpful. The office in Dubai also offers continuing education programs via satellite to health care professionals in the region.

Siebens retired in 1959 at age fifty-four and turned over the Siebens Oil Company to his son, William, who had just received his degree in petroleum engineering. To keep his children interested in pursuing careers despite their inheritance, Siebens told me he set up rewards for academic performance—so much money for an A, three-quarters of that amount for a B, half for a C, and nothing for a D. And what of the inheritance when the child marries? "We have a special committee of family members for that," he confided. "If they approve of the prospective partner, they tell the family member they will get $1 million a year, starting at age forty. If they disapprove, they tell the family member they will not get the money." Why age forty? "By the time they get to forty you have a good idea of their character and how they're going to behave."

One of the chief beneficiaries of Siebens's philanthropy was Buena Vista College in Storm Lake, Iowa, to which he gave $18 million to establish the Harold Walter Siebens School of Business/Siebens Forum to honor his father, an alumnus. I spoke at the school's dedication on October 3, 1985: "Private giving for public purposes is great, powerful, and a unique American tradition. Today, facilities such as these have been made possible solely as a consequence of free enterprise as demonstrated so admirably by the career of Harold Siebens."

At about the same time Siebens made his gift for the business school, the red-brick building that had housed Mayo's group practice since 1914 had to be demolished for safety reasons. The site was ideal for consolidating Mayo educational activities (including the Mayo Alumni Center) and thus for bringing a new cohesiveness to one component of the Mayo triad of medical care, medical education, and medical research. Knowing how responsive Siebens was to entrepreneurship, Keith G. Briscoe, president of Buena Vista College, encouraged us to discuss our needs with the philanthropist. Our pitch to Siebens was that a gift to Mayo for a much-needed educational building might allow some of the graduates at Mayo to become movers and shakers!

We shared several designs with Siebens for the new fourteen-story building, which would adjoin the 1928 Plummer Building, and we finally settled on one from Hammel, Green, and Abrahamson of Minneapolis. Siebens was in Toronto when the planning reached the late stages, and he invited me to show him the architect's model there so he could have a look before making a final decision. I booked a first-class reservation so I would have room to place the model in the seat next to me, which I did, with the flight attendant's kind permission. Canadian customs officials were not so accommodating. Wondering whether I was trying to get money from a Canadian citizen for this building, they took me and the model to an office and interviewed me for about an hour before finally deciding I could enter Canada with the model. My meeting with Siebens and his wife, Estelle, was much more cordial!

Siebens agreed to provide half the cost of the proposed new building, with other Mayo benefactors matching his philanthropy. One condition was that the entire amount be pledged before groundbreaking. Jay and Rose Phillips of Minneapolis provided funds for a four-hundred-seat hall, the largest meeting room on the Mayo Rochester campus. Its teleconference capabilities enable Mayo to send and receive seminars to and from remote sites. Mary Lou and Judd C. Leighton provided funds for a state-of-the-art auditorium with both a personal gift and support from the Leighton-Oare Foundation. Glenn and Norma Hanssen Hage gave funds for the Hage Atrium, whose splendid staircase enhances the area connecting the Siebens Building under the street to the Mayo Building.

Between the grand stairway and the patient cafeteria is a seven-foot bronze figure by French sculptor Auguste Rodin. In the fourteenth century, King Edward III of England ordered six citizens of Calais, France, to surrender the keys of the city. They volunteered to be martyred so that other citizens would be spared. The English spared the six burghers as well, and the city of Calais commissioned Rodin to commemorate them. The Fran and Ray Stark Foundation presented the figure of one of these, *Jean d'Aire,* to Mayo to honor Mayo physician E. Rolland Dickson, chair of the board of development. Ray Stark, a noted film producer from the golden age of Hollywood, was a loyal patient of Mayo. Busts of Harold and Estelle Siebens that appear at the entrance of the building were sculpted by Felix de Weledon, who also created the Walter Siebens bust at Buena Vista College.

Harold Siebens died at his home in the Bahamas in January 1989 before Mayo formally opened the Siebens Building in October of that year. Funding from his foundation enables Mayo to support new research activities in molecular medicine, so important for determining the genetic basis of diseases and thus their prevention and cure.

visiting the Johnson Ranch

The board of development decided that several of its members should visit former president Lyndon Johnson at his ranch. Might he make a donation to Mayo? This followed Johnson's stepping down from Mayo's board of trustees, not long before his death on January 22, 1973.

Three members—neurologist and development chair Kendall Corbin, board of governors chair Emmerson Ward, and I—went to LBJ's ranch. He met our plane (provided by Atherton Bean) at his private landing strip, piled us into his car, and off we went, chasing longhorn cattle and deer. As the car bounced in every direction, Johnson confided that he was test-driving it. Corbin, who had a sore back due to a lumbar disc, was in agony the whole time. We arrived at Johnson's ranch in time for lunch, after which he took us on a walking tour to see his proposed burial site. On the way, we walked through the recently opened Johnson Museum, pausing to use the restroom—the first and only time I have used a urinal standing next to a former president of the United States!

When we returned to Johnson's house, I outlined for him Mayo's plans for studies on atherosclerosis and the need for supporting research in lipid metabolism. Johnson in turn told us of his attempts to raise $35 million for the LBJ School of Public Affairs at the University of Texas. He had given $1.5 million, along with earnings from his 1971 memoirs, *The Vantage Point: Perspectives of the Presidency, 1963–1969.* One friend had donated $1 million toward the school, another friend $500,000, but that was it. While our visit undoubtedly increased Johnson's goodwill toward us, being $32 million short in Texas precluded his giving anything to Mayo.

Barbara Woodward Lips

Mayo's single most generous benefactor was Barbara Woodward Lips of San Antonio, Texas, a patient at the clinic for some four decades. Her husband, Charles Storch Lips, was a successful lawyer who had invested wisely in land, oil, and stocks. She first came to Rochester in 1952 a few years after they had married.

Barbara Lips gave $100,000 to Mayo Foundation for research in Parkinson's disease, and, after her husband's death in 1970, she provided funds for the

Charles Storch Lips Memorial Laboratory for Neurochemistry. She made many additional gifts to the clinic during her lifetime, and developed close friendships with her physicians at Mayo. She also seemed to enjoy visiting one-on-one with development staff and seeing firsthand the spaces where her funds would be used. In outlining guidelines for the development of space with her gifts she was both forthright and diplomatic. I met her many times while I was development chair at Mayo. Once, after we visited an area in the Charlton Building being developed as a patient waiting area, she wrote me with specific color choices, consonant with her southwestern tastes. Although Mayo reserves the right to select such details according to overall needs, the interior decorating staff were able to use her colors in the upholstery and other aspects in the spacious area. Mayo honored Barbara Woodward Lips in 1989 by naming the atrium in the Charlton Building for her. The atrium, which extends from the subway level to the fourth floor, features a waterfall cascading over a granite outcropping to a pool below, a design inspired by Lake Superior's North Shore.

After her death in March 1995, Barbara Woodward Lips bequeathed $127.9 million to the Mayo Foundation, the largest gift to an academic medical center in American history. Confident that the Mayo Foundation would identify the most important priorities for her generosity, she placed no restrictions on the use of this gift. In her honor, the Mayo board of trustees created the Barbara Woodward Lips Endowment for Translational Research. Six priority areas within the clinic's broad research activities benefit from the Lips money: molecular medicine, malignant diseases, organ transplantation, cardiovascular diseases, neurodegenerative diseases, and childhood diseases. Mayo also named three professorships in her honor.

Bruce and Ruth Rappaport

I first met Bruce Rappaport in 1976 when I was dean of Mayo Medical School. A mutual friend, David Barzilai, an endocrinologist and Mayo alumnus, brought us together when Barzilai was dean of Haifa Medical School. At that time, he wanted Rappaport, a former classmate as well as board chair of the Bank of New York and chair of Inter Maritime Bank in Geneva, to help fund a research institution in association with the medical school. Barzilai believed such an institute would enhance the interchange of the medical scientists with the clinical faculty in Rambam Hospital, the teaching hospital associated with the medical school. Rappaport was interested in the proposal but wanted a second opinion, and Barzilai suggested me. I told Rappaport that I thought the plan was outstanding, and he and his wife, Ruth, funded the Rappaport Family Institute for Research in the Medical

Sciences at the Technion-Israel Institute of Technology, which opened in 1979 with Rappaport as board chair.

From its beginning, I have been a member of the Rappaport Family Institute's scientific advisory board. It has been served by several outstanding chairs, including Michael Sela of the Weizmann Institute of Science in Rehovat and Matthew Scharff of the Albert Einstein School of Medicine of Yeshiva University in New York. The institute's distinguished directors have included Israeli scientist Yoram Palti of Carmel Biosensors and Aaron J. Cichanover of the Technion-Israel Institute of Technology. The 2000 recipients of the Albert Lasker Award for Basic Medical Research included two researchers from the Rappaport Family Institute: former director Aaron Cichanover and his colleague Avram Hershko, who shared the award with Alexander Varshavsky of the California Institute of Technology in Pasadena. The award recognized their joint discovery of a small protein, ubiquitin, which plays a key role in regulating cell growth and division, as well as the role of cells in immunity, inflammation, and cancer (such as cancer of the cervix).

The Rappaports also provided substantial funds to the Haifa Medical School, whose Bruce Rappaport Faculty of Medicine reported in 2001 that it had coaxed stem cells into producing insulin in tissue culture. This finding could one day lead to a treatment for Type I diabetes. The Rappaports also established the American-Technion Program for qualified American citizens and permanent residents of the United States. Conducted in English, the program is a four-year program leading to the M.D. degree from the Technion-Israel Institute of Technology–Bruce Rappaport Faculty of Medicine.

The Rappaports have likewise been generous with gifts to the Mayo Foundation, which invited them to "Rappaport Day at Mayo" on October 31, 1983. For Mayo, the event was a long-awaited opportunity to thank them directly for establishing the Clinician-Investigator Fellowships. At a reception and dinner for them at Mayo Foundation House, I presented the eleven scholars to the Rappaports. The fellows came from a broad range of the medical and surgical specialties in the Mayo Graduate School. (Mayo president and CEO Michael B. Wood was a Rappaport scholar, as was Mayo's director for research, John Burnett Jr.) The evening was a success but for one false note. During the reception, as I was talking with Ruth Rappaport, Bruce rushed into the room and shouted, "Do you hear that? They're playing the German national anthem!" The string quartet we had hired was playing Hayden's "Emperor Quartet," originally written for the emperor of Austria and then adopted by Germany as its national anthem in 1922. Banned at the end of World War II, it was readopted with new lyrics by

West Germany in 1950. Its association with the country that had perpetrated the Holocaust was too painful for the Rappaports to bear. At my request, the quartet played a more appropriate piece.

In addition, the Rappaports provided funds for a joint research project on cardiovascular biology involving the Rappaport Institute and the Mayo Clinic and Foundation. The first Rappaport Mayo symposium, "Recent Advances in Research on Cardiovascular Diseases," took place in 1997 at the Rappaport Family Institute in Haifa. The second, "Therapeutic Horizons in Cardiovascular Disease," in 1999 was at the Mayo Clinic in Rochester.

I cherish my long years of friendship with the Rappaports, who are as generous personally as they are philanthropically. In 1997, for instance, when we met at a scientific meeting in Scotland of representatives of the Rappaport Institute and colleagues from the medical school at Dundee, Bruce invited my wife and I to stay at his home in London's Grosvenor House on our return trip through England. He instructed us to have all our meals served in the apartment's dining room by the hotel chef, but we decided instead to eat in the hotel dining room so he would not have to pay for our meals. We were eating breakfast the morning after our arrival when I was paged for a phone call. Bruce was calling from Geneva. Why had we not done what he said?

Leslie and Susan Gonda

Mayo opened the Gonda Building, the largest construction project in its history, in October 2001. Leslie and Susan Gonda, for whom the building is named, were natives of Hungary who survived the Holocaust. Leslie Gonda, born Leslie Goldschmïed, changed his name to Gonda after escaping from a Nazi labor camp; Susan Neufeld was liberated from Auschwitz by the Allies in 1945. The two met in Budapest, married in Switzerland, and built a succession of successful businesses in Venezuela before moving to California with their three children. With his son, Louis, and a friend, Steven Udvar-Hazy, Gonda created International Lease Finance Corporation, one of the largest aircraft-leasing firms in the world. In 2002, *Forbes* magazine named both Leslie and Louis Gonda to its list of the 400 Richest Americans.

As longtime Mayo patients, the Gondas developed keen insight and a deep appreciation for the Mayo model of care. They have provided exceptional philanthropic support for state-of-the-art facilities through the Leslie and Susan Gonda (Goldschmïed) Foundation, which honors their family heritage and loved ones lost in the Holocaust. Embodying the spirit of altruism and generosity, they established Mayo's Gonda Vascular Center at Mayo in 1992, the first of its kind in the world, within the Eisenberg Building of Methodist Hospital. Their commitment brings to life a proverb that Leslie Gonda often quotes: "If the great oak doesn't grow, it will die."

The Gonda Foundation provided a $45 million gift for the first phase (ten floors and subway) of the Gonda Building, which broke ground in 1998 as the largest construction project in Mayo history. It occupies the site where the Damon Hotel once stood. (The hotel, whose name honored Hattie May Damon Mayo, the wife of William J. Mayo, was for a few years a hospital. Whenever I think of the Damon Hospital, I recall the remark of a Mayo medical consultant: "What this place needs is a board-certified arsonist.") Louis Gonda and his wife, Kelly, joined Leslie and Susan Gonda as the lead donors of the building's second phase, which extends it to twenty floors. Patients, alumni, Mayo staff, and other philanthropies have since joined the Gondas, contributing some $200 million toward construction.

Architect John Waugh, the son and grandson of Mayo physicians, designed the Gonda Building in consultation with architect Cesar Pelli through Ellerbe Beckett of Minneapolis, the firm that constructed the first Mayo building in 1914. The Gonda Building further integrates Mayo's medical specialties by joining the Mayo Building on the south and the Charlton Building of Rochester Methodist Hospital on the north. Bridging outpatient examination areas and inpatient hospital services, it forms the largest interconnected medical facility of its kind in the world. When all twenty floors (including the subway) are completed, the $375 million building will add 1.625 million square feet of space to the Mayo campus. (By contrast, the Mayo Building has a total of 1.1 million square feet of space.) Mayo has established a move-in schedule for the first ten floors that will continue through 2003. Ten more stories can be added to the building in the future, bringing the total to thirty stories, if more space is needed.

The David Geffen Auditorium in the subway of the Gonda Building has tiered seating for more than two hundred guests and three-way video-conferencing capability that allows staff at the Rochester clinic to connect with colleagues in Jacksonville and Scottsdale. In the subway is the Nathan Landow Atrium, a glass wall 360 feet long and fifty feet tall looking on the Siebens Medical Education and Plummer Buildings. In the Landow Atrium is the twenty-eight-foot-tall *Man and Freedom* sculpture that previously hung on the north exterior of the Mayo Building. Serena Fleischhaker donated the thirteen spectacular chandeliers that hang over the building's west subway.

Mayo's experience in the transplantation of organs and tissues illustrates the importance of integrating medical specialties to provide better care to patients who must see many specialists in different locations. With completion of the Gonda Building, all transplant-related practices will be consolidated so that specialists may collaborate to meet the needs of their patients—such as when Mayo surgeons performed the nation's first heart/lung/liver transplant in 1996. In addition, Mayo has developed a program for the synergy of practice, research, and education in advancing the care of patients requiring transplantation.

Mayo has been the beneficiary of a legacy of goodwill handed down through generations of compassionate care. William J. Mayo described medicine in 1910 as "a cooperative science—the clinician, the specialist, and the laboratory workers uniting for the good of the patient." In 2002 alone, fifty-six thousand donors had made gifts totaling $121 million to the Mayo Foundation. Everyone involved—trustees, physicians, administrators, alumni, and the men and women of the development section—can share in the pride of Mayo Medical School, the new buildings and facilities, the endowed professorships, and the educational and research programs strengthened by the generosity of Mayo's benefactors.

In the fall of 1986, near the end of my service as chair and director for development at Mayo, I set off for Japan to lecture on my research on the vascular system. Soon, however, I received an urgent message from my wife, Helen. Her doctor had found an unsuspected ovarian cancer and she needed surgery immediately. The months that followed were the saddest of my life.

8 Transitions

Much has happened at the Mayo Clinic since I first read about it in The Doctors Mayo *during that summer of 1946 – the year Helen and I celebrated our first wedding anniversary. Professionally and personally, much has happened to me as well, and until 1987 Helen was by my side, sharing and celebrating with me all of my successes and accomplishments. But that year, after four wonderful decades together, I lost Helen to cancer, and I missed her terribly.*

Yet love unexpectedly found me again, and two years later I married Marion Etzwiler, with whom I recently celebrated our fourteenth anniversary. Since my retirement from Mayo in 1990, Marion and I have shared a rich life, blessed by a blended family of six children and thirteen grandchildren. Our travels have taken us as far as New Zealand, where we lived during the summer of 1994 while I was a guest lecturer at the University of Auckland medical school, and back and forth along the roads of Minnesota, where we log the eighty-five miles between our two homes: one in Minneapolis, where Marion maintains an active social and volunteer life, and one in Rochester, where I, as an emeritus Mayo staff member, continue my research interests as chair of the Mayo Committee on the Application of Gene Therapy.

As I look back on my fifty years at the Mayo Clinic and Foundation, I am astonished at its metamorphosis beyond what William Worrall Mayo, and particularly his sons, Charles Horace Mayo and William James Mayo, first envisioned. I am also gratified by my opportunities to play a part in that growth as a researcher, educator, and partner in what is, arguably, the world's greatest medical group practice.

widowed

In the fall of 1986, I set off for Japan to lecture on my research on the vascular system at three medical schools, starting at Shiga University of Medical Sciences. I had just finished the next lecture, at Kyushu University in Fukuoka, when I received an urgent telephone call from Helen. She had been diagnosed with ovarian cancer and was scheduled for immediate surgery. I canceled my last commitment at Yamanashi Medical College and caught the first plane back to Rochester.

Ovarian cancer is difficult to diagnose in its early stages, since it is hidden in the abdominal cavity. There are no symptoms until the disease has advanced. Helen's surgeon found that her cancer had spread to other abdominal organs. She commenced chemotherapy at once, but it did not stop the spread of the malignant tumor.

As we sat and talked in the evenings, we knew that no treatment would be successful, that the outcome was inevitable. Both Helen's parents had died by then, and, as an only child, she regretted she had no sister. Our daughter-in-law, Wendy, with her nursing skills, was of great help and comfort to Helen. My colleague, Maurice J. Martin, then head of the Mayo Department of Psychiatry, was also most supportive to Helen, both at the clinic and later during visits to her at our condominium. Her physicians put her on steroids, which helped to maintain her strength.

In her brave way, Helen decided we should make a final visit to our relatives in Northern Ireland so that she could say good-bye. Our daughter, Gillian, and our son, Roger, then a medical resident in the Mayo Graduate School of Medicine, together with Wendy, accompanied us on this sad journey in May 1987. Throughout it all, I marveled at Helen's strength of character. The visit was exhausting for her, and as we drove to the airport for the trip back to Rochester, we knew the end was near. Three months later, in the early afternoon of August 10, Helen died at our home. We had been married for forty-two years.

a new relationship

Months later, after attending a meeting in Washington, D.C., I was in the Northwest Airlines World Club awaiting my flight back to Minnesota. As I went to get a cup of coffee, I noticed the beautiful woman who had just come into the room. I stayed close to the coffee counter, hoping she might like some coffee too. I smiled at her, and she smiled back—but kept walking. Soon the flight was called, and she went to collect her luggage. I followed.

Fortunately for me, her bag was stuck in the luggage rack, and I freed it for her.

The flight was delayed (more good fortune!), and in the next twenty minutes we had time to exchange our life histories. My new acquaintance was Marion Etzwiler, president of the Minneapolis Foundation, a major philanthropic organization in Minnesota since 1915. Marion was involved in raising private funds and deciding how best to allocate the money in the community. I explained to her my role as chair of the Mayo board of development. She told me about her impending divorce, that she was an only child who had done much of her growing up in Indiana, and that she was the mother of four children, three daughters and a son. I told her that my wife had recently died of cancer, and that I had a daughter and a son.

Marion and I discovered that we also had a Mayo connection. In the 1920s her father, George Armitage Grassby, consulted with Henry Plummer in designing a pneumatic-tube system to carry patients' records from place to place. A mechanical engineer and inventor, Grassby had invented the pulley system found in many dry goods stores in the 1930s, 1940s, and 1950s. With Grassby's system, a clerk placed money in a cage attached to the pulley, pulled a chain, and sent it up to the cashier, who made change, then sent the cage back to the clerk. The pneumatic system that Grassby and Plummer designed some seventy-five years ago is still in use today at Mayo.

My chance meeting with Marion marked the beginning of our courtship. (She likes to remind me that I was in first class while she had a ticket in coach; her children like to tease me that I picked her up at the Washington airport.) Our families all liked one another and supported us when we announced our marriage plans. With all of our children and grandchildren in attendance, Marion and I were wed in her church, Westminster Presbyterian in Minneapolis, on April 22, 1989.

A dramatic event early in our married life occurred in New York City during a visit to my daughter, Gillian. On a sunny October day, Marion suggested we take the Circle Line cruise around Manhattan to see Ellis Island, the Statue of Liberty, and the New York skyline. Hardly had the boat entered the Harlem River when Marion told me that a man four rows ahead of us seemed ill and she suggested I check on him. By the time I moved forward he had fallen off his chair—he had been shot through the back and shoulder by a sniper on the shore! I quickly ascertained that the bullet had missed his heart and major arteries, and the boat docked in the South Bronx to permit emergency technicians and police officers to board, while police helicopters flew low over the site from where the shots were fired. The man's family, German tourists on vacation in New York, were stunned.

As a practical matter, the boat would not return to its berth in Manhattan for some time. Since Marion had a late afternoon meeting scheduled in the city, and I had a flight to catch back to Minnesota, we petitioned the captain to let us disembark. The next day, the front page of the *New York Post* carried a picture of Marion and me standing on the deck of the boat! In the aftermath, the German consul in New York visited the victim in the hospital, and Mayor David Dinkins offered to him and his family a personal tour of the city in a bulletproof limousine as soon as the patient had recovered. The German tourist declined the offer in favor of returning home as soon as possible—and Marion has never been able to persuade me to try the Circle Line again.

joining Mayo's emeritus staff

When W. Eugene Mayberry, chair of the Mayo board of governors, asked me to chair the board of development, I told him he should succeed me when the time came for a change in his responsibilities. This occurred when I was sixty-eight, and Mayberry persuaded me to continue my research until I was seventy.

At that time—1990—I became a member of the Mayo emeritus staff, which has offices on the tenth floor of the Plummer Building. Henry Plummer planned this distinctive building, and during its construction Will Mayo telegraphed him from England, saying, "Add a tower; I've bought some bells!" Townsfolk once called the building "Plummer's folly," since they assumed its size was far too great for the number of patients who would come to a small town. How wrong they were! The 1928 Plummer Building helped establish Mayo as an international medical center. I particularly like the eye-level carving on the front of the building showing Henry Plummer perusing plans for its construction. The carving shows an owl, a fitting symbol of Plummer's wise vision of the efficient group practice of medicine.

genetics, genomics, and gene therapy

Medicine has come a long way in the nearly half century since the American scientist James D. Watson and his English colleague Francis H. C. Crick discovered the double helix structure of deoxyribonucleic acid, or DNA. This breakthrough explained how genes work in cells to convey the codes that enable proteins—the chemical workhorses of cells—to make a body grow and function. "We have discovered the secret of life," declared Watson and Crick. (When they received the Nobel Prize in physiology or medicine in

Stockholm in 1992, shared with Maurice Wilkins, Watson is also said to have remarked, "Wouldn't it be great if this discovery could be used to cure human stupidity!")

We at Mayo continue to prepare for the new horizon in medicine—of medical genetics, genomics, and gene therapy. This includes the study of the proteome, the entire protein complement of the genome, which contains the totality of genetic information about the human body. The body has some 25,000 to 35,000 genes, which might encode 100,000 to 200,000 proteins. Already we know that proteins are involved in every aspect of the function of cells and control each regulatory mechanism. Disease modifies the normal functioning and production of proteins.

Unraveling the human genome will have "unprecedented impact and long-lasting value for basic biology, biomedical research, biotechnology, and health care," wrote Francis Collins, head of the National Human Genome Research Institute, in *Science* in 1998. The overwhelming knowledge amassed by the Human Genome Project will provide a greater understanding of the mechanisms underlying human disease—and of the natural genetic variations in humans—than we have ever had. This knowledge is such a precious scientific resource that it must be totally and freely accessible to all scientists, whose research will eventually lead to medical achievements we cannot imagine.

Such genetic research will improve diagnosis and therefore treatment. Collins cites, for example, the code for BRCA1, a gene linked to breast and ovarian cancers. The code can be put on a silicone chip and used to detect the presence or absence of diseases of the gene in a blood sample. In some cases, this allows treatment before the disease develops.

A new branch of medical science known as pharmacogenetics has already developed. It will create a new era of personalized medicine in which treatment is tailored to an individual's genetic profile. Physicians will genetype their patients to determine treatment. This raises ethical and legal concerns, such as patient safety. As in all human experimentation, the efficacy and possible toxicity of gene therapies must first be tested in animals, including primates, before proceeding to human trials. Patient confidentiality is another critical concern. Congress acted in 1998 to block the possibility that personalized genetic information would be used to deny people health insurance or jobs.

Some have stated that financial walls between science and medical practice in academic centers across the United States threaten a schism between bench and bedside. The barriers emerge as the progression of medical science pushes practicing physicians to learn the language of molecular biologists, and pushes biologists to understand the problems facing practicing physicians. We need more clinician-investigators to bridge the gap. Only they can ensure the bonding of biologists and physicians that will move advances in medical genetics toward patient care. Such bench-to-bedside advances will require increased funding from the National Institutes of Health for molecular scientists and clinician-investigators alike.

general clinical research center

The establishment of general clinical research centers in the United States, including the General Clinical Research Center at Mayo, provides clinician-investigators with the specialized staff, facilities, and resources that permit knowledge generated in the laboratory to be translated into better patient care. Mayo formally established its GCRC at Saint Marys Hospital, with both inpatient and outpatient facilities, in 1971. I was the principal investigator from then until 1976.

The center's activities declined during its second decade, but beginning in 1990, Mayo reorganized and revitalized the programs and developed additional facilities at the adjoining Domitilla Building at Saint Marys Hospital. The National Institutes of Health had funded Mayo's GCRC from its founding, but the center's revitalization helped secure competitive renewals of NIH funding in 1994 and 1999. An NIH review panel in 1999 gave Mayo's GCRC an outstanding priority score and recommended full funding for five years of $3 million a year—an action that reflects the number of excellent scientific protocols proposed by clinician-investigators and the continued willingness of volunteers to participate in GCRC studies. Over the past several years, in fact, Mayo's GCRC received biomedical grants for more than two hundred active protocols, more than any other unit in the clinic. The grants include money to train future clinician-investigators. In addition, the GCRC also secured a $4.95 million grant from the Grainger Foundation in September 1997.

Mayo opened an outpatient GCRC in December 1999 on the seventh floor of the Charlton Building in Rochester to facilitate outpatient clinical research and to complement the research facility at Saint Marys Hospital. The new unit boasts state-of-the-art facilities that have the ability and flexibility to adapt to new technologies in medicine. The downtown activities are part of the comprehensive research, education, and clinical training program for new and developing clinician-investigators at Mayo.

Much of the credit for the success of the center's reorganization goes to B. Lawrence Riggs, who served as GCRC director from 1991 through 2001 and with whom I worked as a consultant between 1992 and 1994 to ensure that the proposed activities for the center would be competitive for continued NIH support. A pioneer in the field of osteoporosis, Riggs introduced and applied the first densitometer to measure bone mineral density in the hip and spine. He was the first to define the effects of estrogen on bone remodeling in osteoporosis. With Mayo biochemist Thomas Spelsberg and others, he demonstrated estrogen receptors in bone cells and showed that estrogen plays a major role in bone loss. I nominated Riggs for a Mayo Distinguished Alumnus Award, which he received in May 2001. He is the Purvis and Roberta Tabor Professor of Medical Research at Mayo Medical School, as well as former chair of the Mayo Division of Endocrinology and Metabolism.

Future goals for Mayo's GCRC include developing core facilities for genomics and proteonomics (functions of all the proteins); integrating cutting-edge technologies such as stem-cell therapy, gene therapy, and xenotransplantation; and developing educational activities at the Mayo Clinics in Jacksonville and Scottsdale.

Mayo and medicine's new horizon

Upon completion of the Human Genome Project in 2000, the Mayo Rochester Research Strategic Issues Committee formed the Genomics Task Force to survey the status of genomic research at the Mayo Clinic in Rochester and to advise how Mayo should respond to developments. The same year, 2000, the Mayo Rochester Education Committee named Thomas Spelsberg of the Department of Biochemistry and Molecular Biology as director for genome education. Spelsberg organized the Genomics Education Steering Committee to plan and develop an education program for physicians and allied health workers in this new area of medicine. This involves identifying all the genes involved in each human disease and using this information in diagnosis, prognosis, and treatment, as well as assessing predisposition to each disease. The board of governors of Mayo Rochester approved using funds from the George M. Eisenberg Foundation and the Mayo Foundation for this important effort.

Understanding medical genomics will involve knowledge in the related sciences of bioinformatics, proteomics (computer-based determination of protein functions), and pharmacogenetics/pharmacogenomics (development of new drugs targeted to newly discovered genes and their proteins). This new medicine will allow scientists to identify human genes and their protein products and understand how they function, and thus to develop new laboratory tests and personalized therapies for genetically diagnosed diseases.

Upon the recommendation of the Genomics Education Steering Committee, Mayo in 2001 formally established the Genomics Research Center. Under the direction of Richard Weinshilboum, chair of the Department of Molecular Pharmacology and Experimental Therapeutics at Mayo Rochester, the new center will foster research-related genomics activities. This will include establishing a translational genomics laboratory available to all staff. Mayo has authorized three new staff positions to oversee the laboratory, strengthen laboratory-based genomics research, and establish a bioinformatics infrastructure.

For one of these positions, director of the molecular medicine program, Mayo recruited Stephen Russel, a hematologist who headed the gene therapy group at the Medical Research Council in Cambridge, England, the British equivalent of the National Institutes of Health. Russel points out that diseases arising from single gene defects are potential candidates for therapies in which the correct genes can be injected into cells to change the cells' behavior. Another type of gene therapy—with obvious applications for cancer patients—involves injecting proteins into cells that either kill the cells or cause them to be sensitive to drugs that kill the cells.

There is today a shortage of medical geneticists. Based on Mayo's plans, the NIH has established the Faculty Development Award for Genetics in Medicine at the Mayo Clinic in Scottsdale. But future development of the Mayo Genomics Research Center may require $80 million to recruit additional staff and provide research facilities for them. Another important clinical problem is obtaining compatible human donor organs to replace diseased kidneys, hearts, lungs, livers, and pancreases. Demand far exceeds supply. Mayo has a major xenotransplantation research program under way that may resolve this problem. In essence, molecular biologists and transplant surgeons are investigating the possibility that genetically modified organs from pigs might be transplanted into humans as replacements for their own diseased organs.

genomic research: relationships with industry

For centralized, shared genomic research to succeed, Mayo must establish strong relationships with industry. Active, mutually beneficial relationships with industry will enable Mayo investigators and ultimately Mayo's clinical laboratories, staff, and patients to have access to the latest technologies to test research and clinical applications. Such relationships require protecting patient rights and confidentiality with the help of a Mayo medical ethicist, as well as educating staff about the science of genomics so that clinical investigation can benefit both patient and health care provider. Such educational programs are now being developed through the Mayo Rochester Education Committee and will undoubtedly be implemented through Mayo's General Clinical Research Center.

Before engaging with industry, Mayo must develop a clearly articulated plan for negotiations between industrial partners and Mayo Medical Ventures, the Mayo Strategic Alliances Committee, or other appropriate institutional groups. It must also guard against the financial interests of investigators in the biotechnology and pharmaceutical industries that are incompatible with ethical patient experiments. Likewise, as Jeffrey M. Leiden suggested in *Circulation Research,* gene therapy investigators from academic medical centers must not have personal significant relationships with companies that may benefit financially from the results of clinical trials. Mayo's existing policies and guidelines governing relationships with industry already cover such issues as disclosure of private financial interests relevant to a research project and ownership rights to inventions or discoveries, as well as licensure and royalties.

I am excited about the challenges of chairing the newly appointed Mayo Committee on the Application of Gene Therapy. The role of this committee is to review specific protocols proposed by Mayo consultants and to decide which ones merit approval. It submits its recommendations for appropriate action to the Mayo Institutional Review Board, established by federal law to review all proposals for any research in humans. The committee is also responsible to the Institutional Review Board for the continuous monitoring of approved projects, including patient safety and the effectiveness of the therapy.

family life

My marriage to Marion has brought each of us the added blessing of an extended family. Between us, she and I have four daughters, two sons, and six sons- and daughters-in-law. We also have thirteen grandchildren—many birthdays to keep track of!

After completing her studies at Wheaton College, Tufts University, and New York Medical College, my daughter, Gillian, is a clinical associate professor of medicine at Weill Medical College of Cornell University, with a clinical practice in a private office in New York City. She is a past president of the New York Allergy Society and the first elected chair of the American Academy of Allergy, Asthma, and Immunology, the main group for her specialty. With

Gillian as chair, the American Academy of Allergy, Asthma, and Immunology has raised several million dollars for research and teaching. She lectures nationally about drug allergies, her principal research interest.

Gillian's husband, Eduardo Mestre, has degrees from Yale University and Harvard Law School. He practiced general corporate law at Cleary, Gottlieb, Steen and Hamilton before joining Salomon Brothers in New York City in 1977. The company has changed names many times since then; Eduardo is chair of investment banking at Citigroup Global Markets, its current name. He has helped facilitate multiple telecommunications mergers. *Investment Dealers Digest* named him "Banker of the Year" for 1999. Outside of Citigroup, he is chair of the board of the WNYC Foundation, which produces New York City public radio. Eduardo is a sixth-generation Cuban. His father, Goar Mestre, was well known in Cuban and Argentinian radio and television, and received a 1987 Emmy for his contributions to broadcasting. When Fidel Castro ousted the Cuban dictator Fulgencio Batista in 1959, Goar fled Cuba at once, boarding a plane at Havana airport where he was seeing his sons, Eduardo and Roberto, off to prep school in the United States. The Mestres assumed that Alicia Mestre, an Argentine citizen, would be safe, but she too quickly left Cuba with their daughters, Alicia and Ani, when she learned her accounts had been frozen by the Castro government. The family eventually settled in Buenos Aires, the original home of Alicia Mestre. The Mestres lost all of their possessions in Cuba. Eduardo's brother and sisters still live in Argentina with their families.

Two of Gillian's and Eduardo's three children have attended Choate Rosemary Hall, the prep-school alma mater of my son, Roger. Cristina was first, and has since graduated from Duke University. Her brother, Edward, graduated from Choate in June 2003 and now attends Duke. Laura, like her father, went to the Taft School, then graduated from Boston College; she lives and works in New York City.

Roger went from Choate to Lawrence University in Appleton, Wisconsin, then was accepted to Queen's University of Belfast, thus becoming the thirteenth member of the Shepherd family to attend this medical school.

(With the many different medical specialties practiced by members of the family, we could start a Shepherd Clinic! In addition to me and my children, my oldest brother, Harry, was a neuroradiologist, and his wife, Rene, a specialist in genitourinary medicine, both at the Royal Victoria Hospital in Belfast. Their oldest son, Ian, is an eye surgeon at the Borders District Hospital at Melrose, Scotland. Their second son, Richard, is a specialist in chest diseases at Belfast City Hospital. Their daughter, Patricia, is a hematologist at the

University of Edinburgh and Western General Hospital in Edinburgh. My second brother, Fred, was a general practitioner in the small country town of Portglenone, Northern Ireland, where we were born. His oldest son, Allister, a surgeon in the British army, is based in England but assigned at intervals to different parts of the world. His youngest son, Charles, is a pediatrician in County Armagh, Northern Ireland. And finally, Harry Shepherd, my father's older brother, for whom my oldest brother, Harry, is named, practiced medicine in England until his sudden death in 1914, five years before I was born.)

After his graduation from Queen's, Roger was a resident at the Mayo Clinic, where he developed a special interest in the diseases of the blood vessels and high blood pressure. He joined the Mayo medical staff in 1989 in the Vascular Center and the Division of Hypertension and Internal Medicine. He is a fellow of the Society of Vascular Medicine and Biology, the American Society of Hypertension, and the American College of Cardiology.

Roger's wife, the former Wendy Alden, graduated from Viterbo College and is a registered public health nurse. They met during Roger's residency rotation at Saint Marys Hospital, where Wendy was a staff nurse. She is a direct descendant of John Alden, who came to America on the *Mayflower*. As he listened to Wendy relate her family story, Roger commented, "That may be, but we also came over on a boat—the *S.S. America*." Roger and Wendy have two sons, John Roger and Alex.

My family has welcomed Marion's four children. Nancy Etzwiler, an attorney in the office of the general counsel at 3M in Maplewood, Minnesota, oversees the legal affairs of 3M in Latin America and South Africa. She is a graduate of Yale University and the University of Virginia law school. Her husband, Dan O'Neill, is a graduate of St. Benedict's College in Atchison, Kansas, and an investment banker in Minneapolis. They live in Afton, Minnesota, with their daughter, Laura Grey.

Lisa Etzwiler and her husband, Randall Clary, are pediatricians. Lisa also attended Yale University, then Johns Hopkins School of Medicine, while Randall studied at the University of Illinois. Lisa is director of pediatric emergency services of a large community hospital in St. Louis. Randall is head of pediatric otolaryngology at Children's Hospital at Washington University in St. Louis. Lisa and Randall have two daughters, Emily and Sally.

Diane (Dee) Etzwiler, who lives in Eugene, Oregon, is a graduate of Lewis and Clark College and the University of Oregon. An architect, she is married to Rob Thallon, also an architect as well as a tenured professor at the

University of Oregon. Rob trained at the University of California at Berkeley and received his master's degree in architecture from the University of Oregon. They have two children, Carter and Claire.

David Etzwiler and his wife, Sarah Truesdell, live in Edina, Minnesota, where David is director of the Medtronic Foundation. He graduated from Northwestern University and earned a master's degree in public policy from Claremont College in California and a law degree from the University of Minnesota. Sarah completed her doctorate in psychology from the University of Minnesota after graduating from Mount Holyoke College in Massachusetts. She is the former associate director of the Student Counseling Center at the College of St. Catherine in St. Paul. David and Sarah have three sons: identical twins Michael and Ryan, and Dylan.

After a decade as director of the Minneapolis Foundation, Marion retired from the organization in June 1994, the summer we lived in New Zealand, when I was a visiting lecturer at the University of Auckland Medical School. Beginning in 1997 she served for three years as a capital-campaign consultant at the University of Minnesota Foundation.

Marion and I celebrated our fourteenth wedding anniversary in April 2003. Because she is busy with charitable and civic activities in Minneapolis and I have responsibilities at Mayo in Rochester, we maintain condominiums in each city. Our commuting lifestyle gives us the flexibility we need to maintain our interests and responsibilities. The miles that separate us are easy to bridge whenever concerts, the theater, or social occasions beckon. Marion and I have also traveled a great deal—to medical meetings in Belgium, Israel, Italy, Hungary, and Scotland, as well as on vacations to Costa Rica with Marion's daughter Dee and her family; through the Panama Canal with my former research fellow, Tore Strandell, and his wife; and, of course, to Ireland, where, in June 2003, I was privileged to become an honorary fellow of the Royal College of Physicians of Ireland. With Marion, I continue to attend Shepherd family reunions every August in County Donegal in Eire, in the little seaside village of Portnoo—the same spot I've vacationed with family since I was ten years old. In 2003, forty-five family members gathered there, including Dee, Rob, Carter, and Claire.

America's health care system

My fifty-year affiliation with Mayo has given me an insider's look into complex questions about the current American system of health care service and delivery. I am proud that Mayo is committed to helping find the answers.

"A major medical institution [such as Mayo] no longer can be content with rendering superior care to the individual patient who gains admission to its services," said Emmerson Ward at the first Mayo Sponsors Day in 1972. "It must [also] look outside its own walls and lead in developing a system which will provide readily accessible, high quality, efficient, continuing, comprehensive medical care from which no one is barred because of economic or social factors."

As a Mayo trustee, former president Lyndon Johnson predicted in 1970 that the solution to health care lies in "wholehearted involvement at all levels of our society." At the second Mayo Sponsors Day in 1973, Senator Hubert H. Humphrey stressed the need to reorganize the nation's health care system. "In the absence of a comprehensive national health care policy," he warned, "we are unlikely to restrain the rising costs of health care or to make quality care accessible and available to every citizen as a basic right." (A champion of civil rights and social causes, Humphrey had a penchant for long speeches that once prompted his wife, Muriel, to tell him, "Hubert, you don't have to be eternal to be immortal.") His first legislative proposal was for medical care for the aged. Medicare was eventually enacted in 1965, after Humphrey was elected vice president. And in a special bicentennial issue of *The Mayo Alumnus* published July 4, 1976, Senator Walter F. Mondale cited Mayo's pioneering approach to health services through group medicine as one way the United States might organize health care resources for maximum effectiveness.

The preferred alternative to universal health care seems to be managed care, delivered by HMOs, or health maintenance organizations. Yet critics consistently complain that nonmedical administrators control the medical care that patients receive—and that the care is often inadequate. In 2001, in fact, state medical associations in California, Georgia, and Texas filed suit against several large health insurers, alleging they illegally used cost-based criteria to approve or deny claims for payment and offered cash incentives to claims reviewers to deny or limit tests and treatment. In Minnesota, Attorney General Mike Hatch acted in July 2001 to break up Allina Health System, a major health-care provider, because of allegations that Allina wasted millions of dollars on executive perks and consultants and used insurance premiums improperly. In response, the Allina board of directors voted to split the system into two nonprofit entities. One now delivers health care through its system of hospitals and clinics, while the other governs its Medica health plan.

According to former Mayo CEO Robert Waller, the challenge is not to manage the current health care system but to change it—to raise its quality, lower its cost, expand the number of those it serves, and simplify delivery.

In a June 21, 2001, talk to Mayo staff on American health care policy, Waller emphasized five principles of change, all of them compatible with Mayo's traditions: that health care must be patient-centered, that patients need better information and opportunities for shared decision-making, that patients must have the freedom to choose both the provider and the payer, that patients must share in the financial consequences as well as in their own health care, and that competition encourages innovation, which is the foundation of education and research.

Waller chaired the Healthcare Leadership Council, composed of fifty-five chief executive officers from all disciplines within the health care system. He said his colleagues on the council (of which Mayo was a charter member) believe most legislators see national health care as a political issue, not as a solution to what ails America's current system. One objective of the council is cost reduction through improvement, which demands protecting physician-patient relationships across markets and government programs, and among network managers, insurance companies, hospitals, and health care systems.

I believe medical care should be controlled by physicians, not by administrators. The American Medical Association supports this concept and other principles of health care reform, including that all rules must apply to all Americans, that patients must be able to appeal HMO decisions to an independent governing body, and that health-care administrators must be as accountable as physicians should their decisions cause patients harm.

The Mayo model of health-care delivery offers the nation a vision of what we can accomplish in this country. Mayo's challenge is to provide the best care to every patient every day by advancing the medical sciences and by training tomorrow's leaders in medicine. Our responsibility is to ensure Mayo's strength for those who will follow us. We must continue collegial and cooperative staff teamwork, with multispecialty integration, unhurried and comprehensive evaluation, and compassionate care supported by the most advanced, innovative, and therapeutic technology and techniques. We must maintain a scholarly environment of research and education, as well as our cherished principle of physician leadership—a Mayo hallmark that has continued since the days of the Mayo brothers.

In addition, we must maintain our valued professional allied health staff, an integrated medical record, and professional compensation that allows us to focus on quality, not quantity, by removing the possibility of personal gain from the treatment recommendations we make to patients. Since Mayo

Foundation and Saint Marys and Rochester Methodist Hospitals are private nonprofit corporations whose medical staff is that of Mayo Clinic, they form an integrated center offering patients medical expertise supported by extensive programs in education and research. The boards of governors of the Mayo Clinics in Rochester, Jacksonville, and Scottsdale approved eight clinician and research education appointments in 2001. Thomas Berquist, education director for Mayo Foundation, said these appointments—a consequence of financial restraints by government on academic medical centers—ensure that faculty will have time for teaching innovation and faculty development. The high quality of education for Mayo professionals will not be eroded.

a half-century of change

How much has the Mayo Clinic grown since the publication of Helen Clapesattle's *The Doctors Mayo* in 1941?

Back then, one clinic employed 179 staff physicians and scientists. As of December 31, 2002, the three Mayo Clinics of Rochester, Jacksonville, and Scottsdale—each a full-fledged clinical practice that integrates medical education and research for optimal patient care—claimed a combined staff of 2,884 physicians and scientists. In addition, there are 1,905 residents, fellows, and temporary professionals, 690 medical students, and 40,835 allied health staff—46,314 employees altogether! Together the clinics saw 501,019 patients in 2002, and admitted 124,633 patients to its hospitals. In Rochester, Saint Marys Hospital has 1,157 licensed beds and Methodist Hospital, 794. In Jacksonville, St. Luke's Hospital has 289 licensed beds, while in Phoenix, Mayo Clinic Hospital has 205.

The Mayo Health System also has a network of clinics and hospitals in sixty-four communities in Minnesota, Iowa, and Wisconsin. These alliances—with clinics in Albert Lea, Austin, Faribault, Fairmont, Lake City, Mankato, Owatonna, and Wabasha (Minnesota); Decorah and New Hampton (Iowa); and Eau Claire, La Crosse, and Menomonie (Wisconsin)—ensure that patients can be cared for more easily, with the same level of competence, in their hometowns.

Upon viewing the Mayo buildings that emerge from the cornfields surrounding Rochester, a visitor once dubbed the city Oz. Yet since 1941, Rochester has been recognized as a cosmopolitan center with big-city sophistication and small-town warmth, all rolled up in a tidy package of 90,000 residents. In fact, *Money Magazine* recognized Rochester as the second most livable city in America in 1997, the most livable small city in the Midwest in 1998, and the "Best Small City in America" in 1999.

Once in a great while, I think back to that summer of 1946 when my brother gave me *The Doctors Mayo* to read while I vacationed with my family along the northwest coast of Ireland. What luck that Fred should have chosen that particular book. What luck that it should captivate me so thoroughly that I would leave behind all that was familiar to make a new life in a new land. What luck that the road from Belfast should be the road to the great and unique medical center that is Mayo.

What wonderful, magnificent luck.

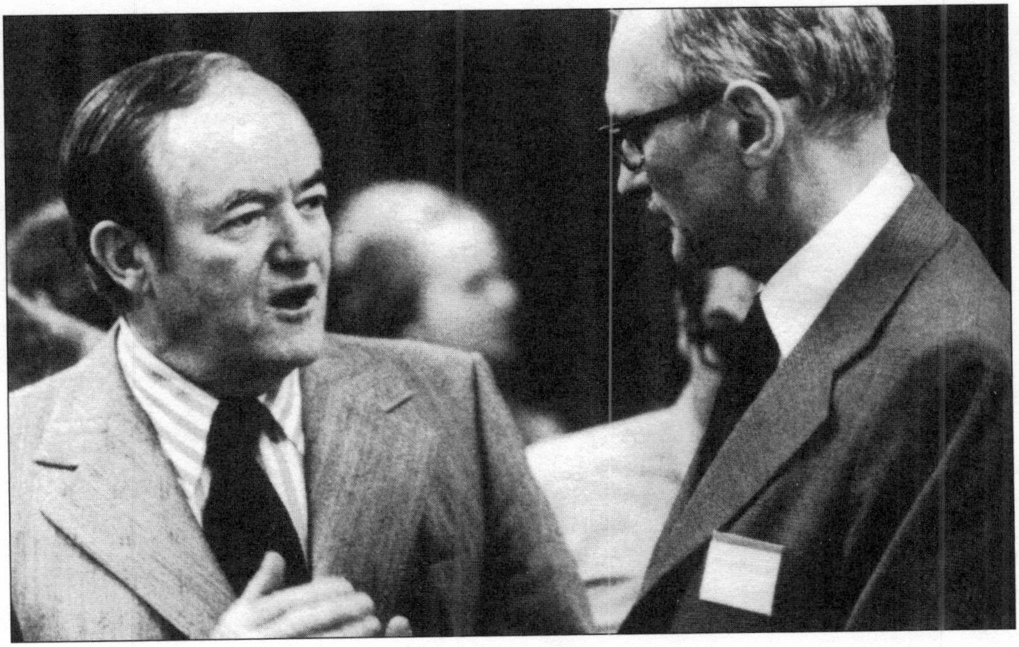

Senator and former vice president Hubert H. Humphrey speaks with me (then Mayo director for research) at the second Mayo Sponsors Day, May 1973. (MAYO PHOTO ARCHIVES)

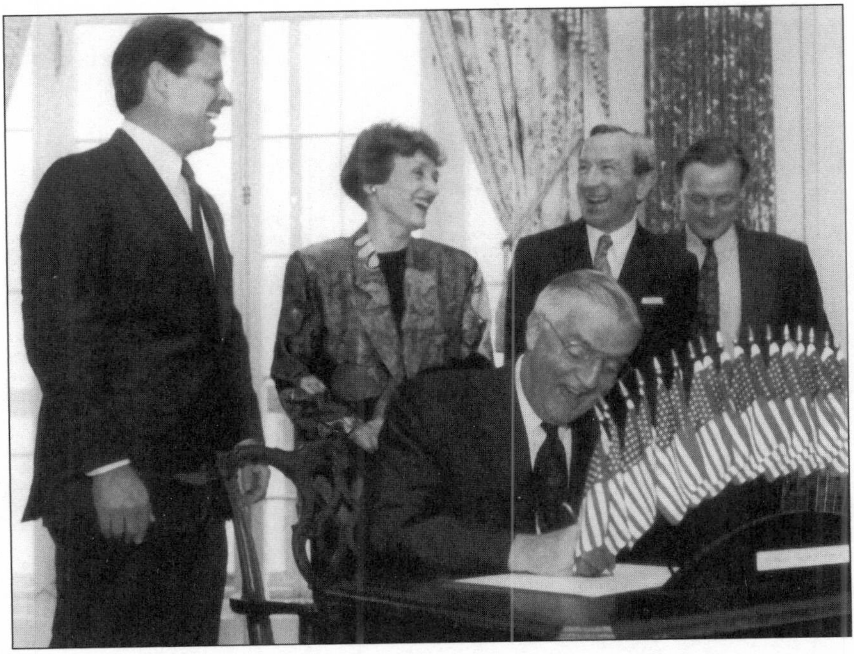

Newly appointed ambassador to Japan and Mayo external trustee Walter F. Mondale (seated) enjoys a hearty laugh as he signs official documents. Standing (from left): Vice President Al Gore, Joan Adams Mondale, Secretary of State Warren Christopher, and Ted Mondale.

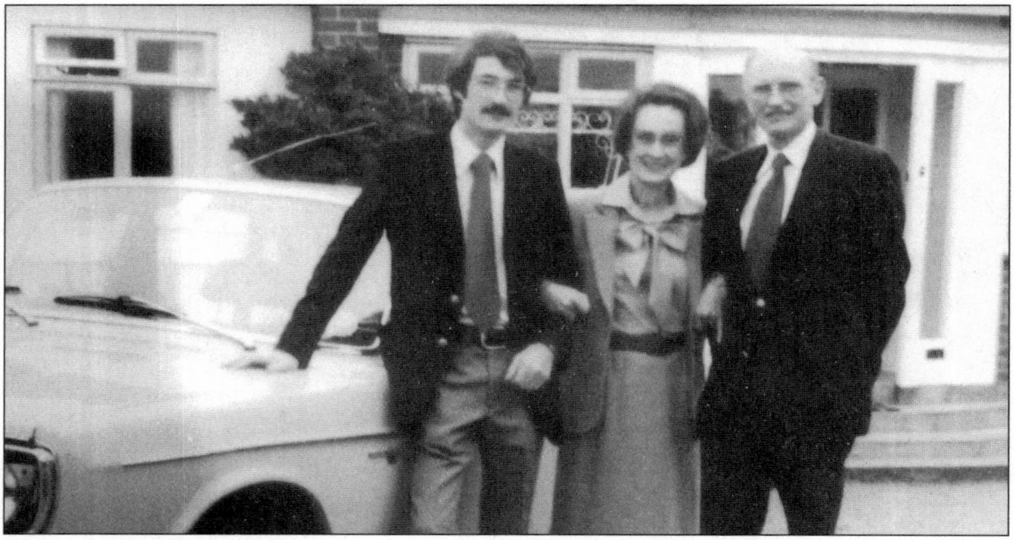

Helen and I with our son, Roger, who became the thirteenth member of the Shepherd family to attend the medical school at Queen's University in Belfast.

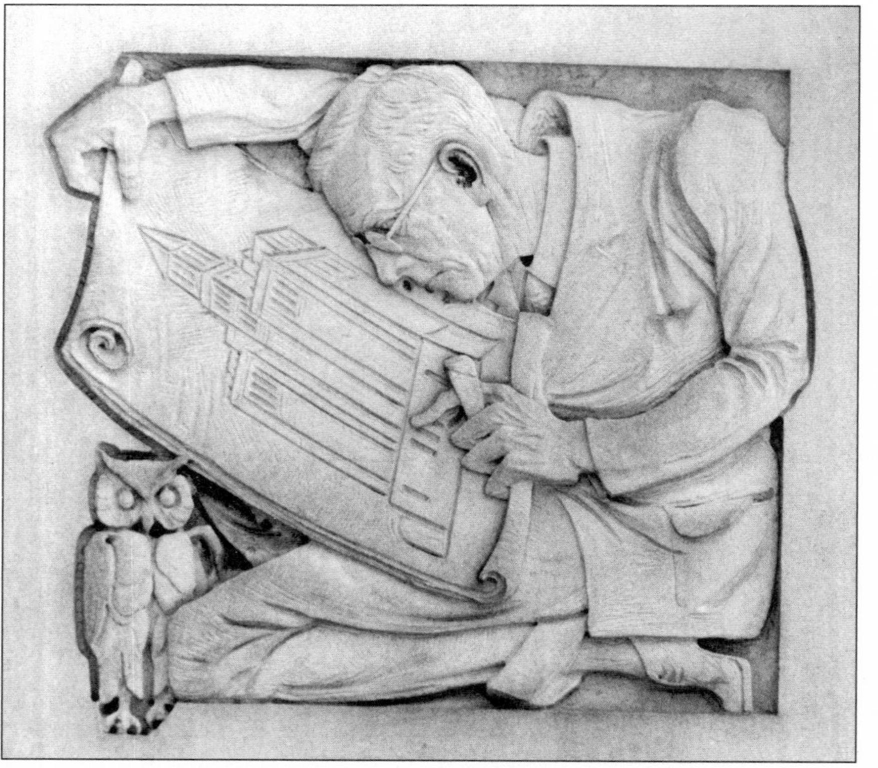

A carving on the west wall of the Plummer Building depicts Henry Plummer planning the building. Note the wise old owl. (MAYO PHOTO ARCHIVES)

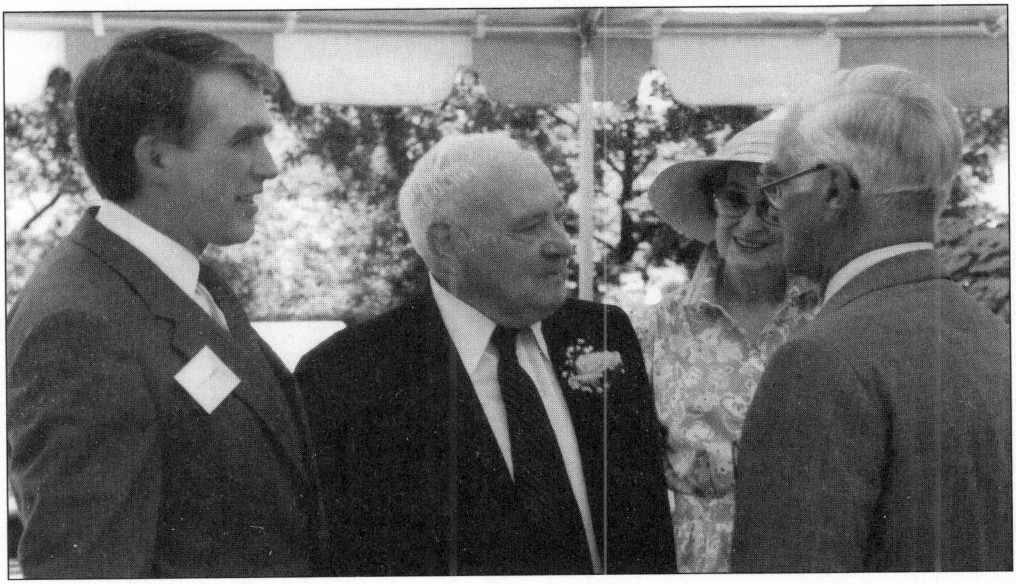

Mayo benefactor George Eisenberg (center) with David Lawrence of the Mayo Development Department (left), Helen Shepherd, and Robert Roesler, chair of Mayo Administration. (MAYO PHOTO ARCHIVES)

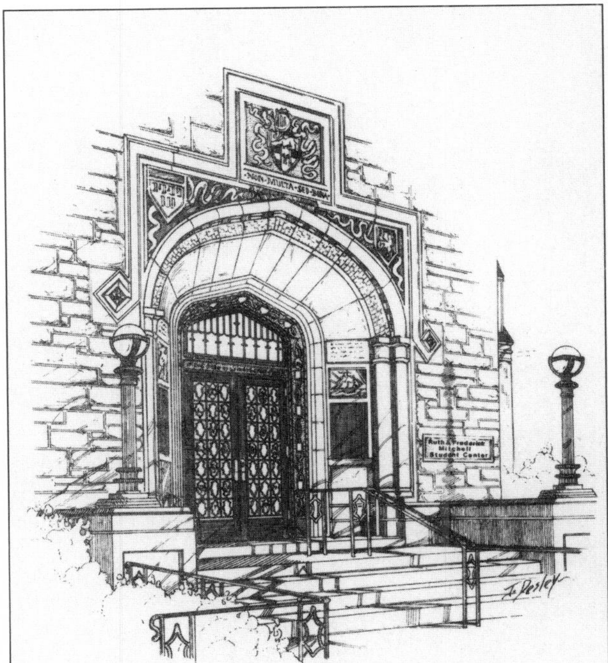

The Ruth and Frederick Mitchell Student Center at Mayo Medical School. (MAYO PHOTO ARCHIVES)

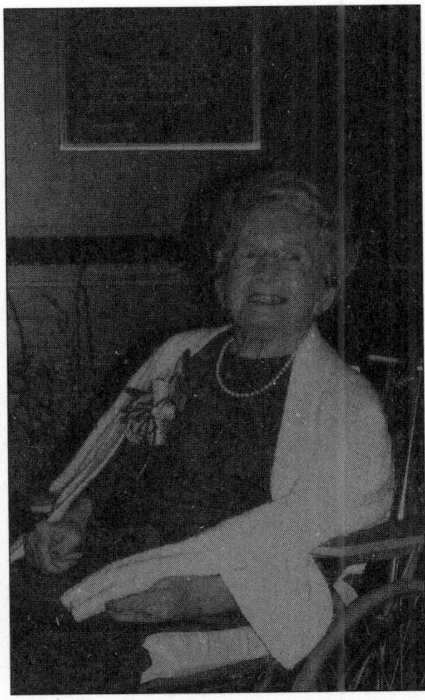

Ruth Charlton Mitchell Masson attends the 1988 opening of the Charlton Building, which adjoins the Eisenberg Building–Rochester Methodist Hospital. (MAYO PHOTO ARCHIVES)

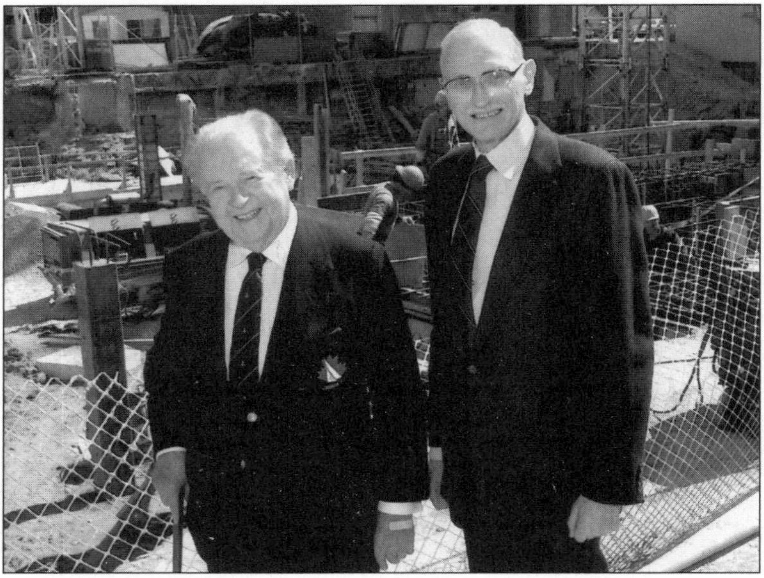

Harold Siebens (left) and I survey the construction site of the Siebens Educational Building. (MAYO PHOTO ARCHIVES)

The Siebens Building (left) was the first at Mayo built entirely with private contributions. (MAYO PHOTO ARCHIVES)

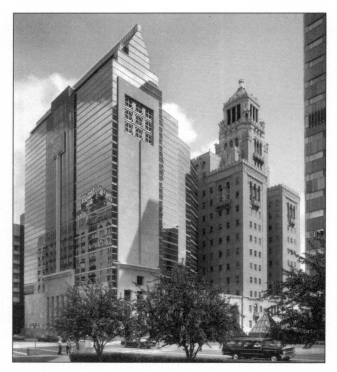

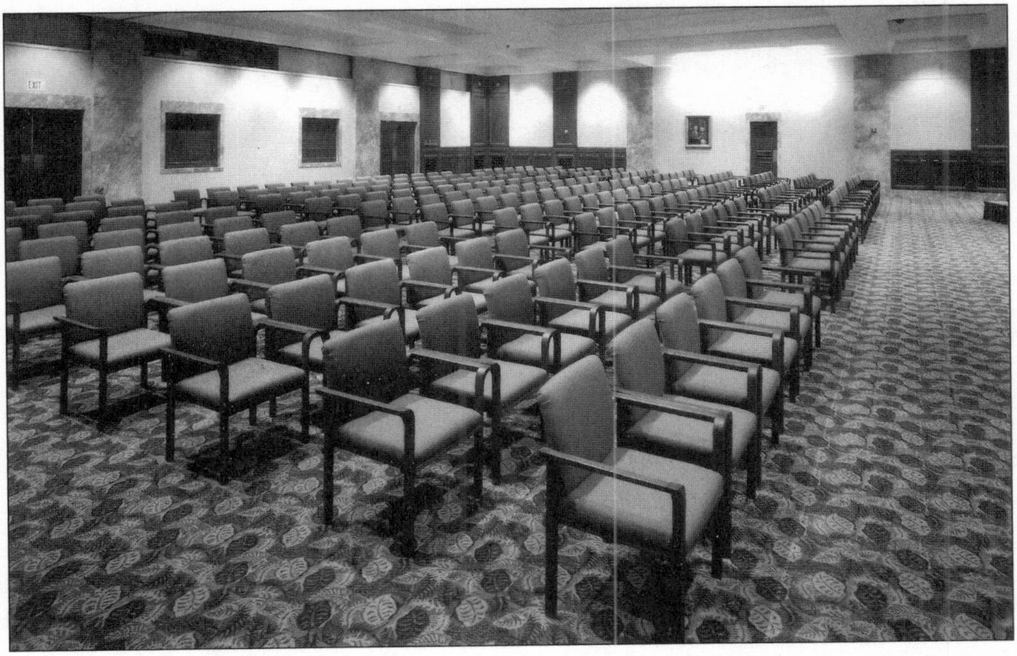

Funds for the Phillips Hall, located on the first floor of the Siebens Building, were provided by Jay and Rose Phillips of Minneapolis. (MAYO PHOTO ARCHIVES)

The Hage Atrium in the Siebens Building was built with funds from Glenn and Norma Hanssen Hage. (MAYO PHOTO ARCHIVES)

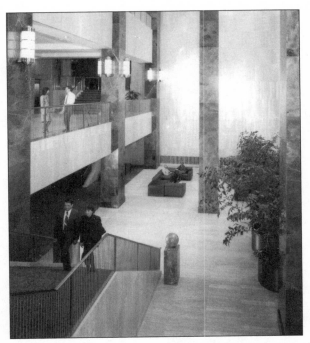

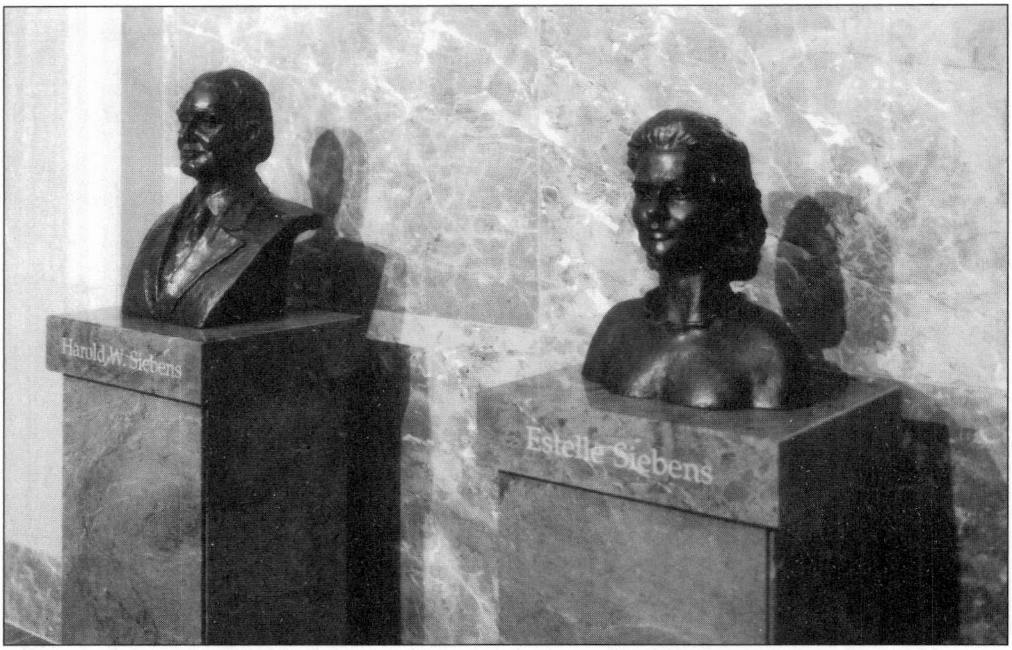

The busts of Harold and Estelle Siebens in the main entrance to the Harold W. Siebens Education Building. (MAYO PHOTO ARCHIVES)

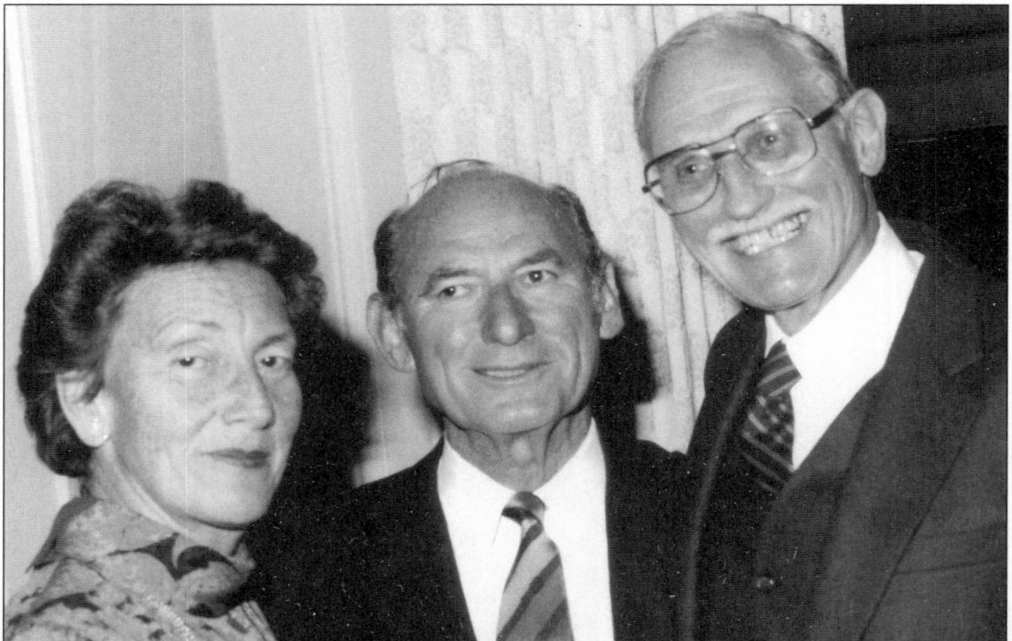

Mayo philanthropists Ruth and Bruce Rappaport with the author. (MAYO PHOTO ARCHIVES)

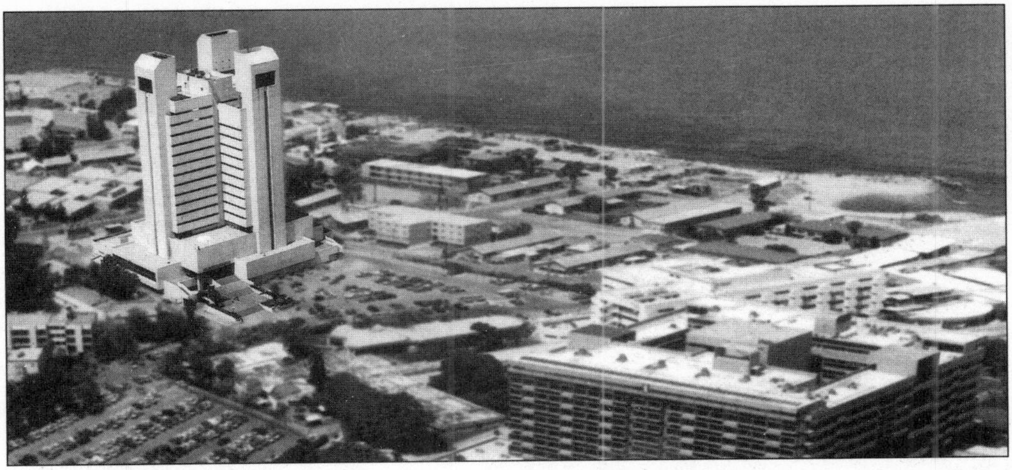

The high-rise Rappaport Family Institute for Research in the Medical Sciences (top left) in Haifa, Israel. The Rambam Hospital is in front on the right, with the Mediterranean Sea in the background.

Aaron Cichanover, director of the Rappaport Family Institute for Research in the Medical Sciences in Haifa, Israel, with the author. (MAYO PHOTO ARCHIVES)

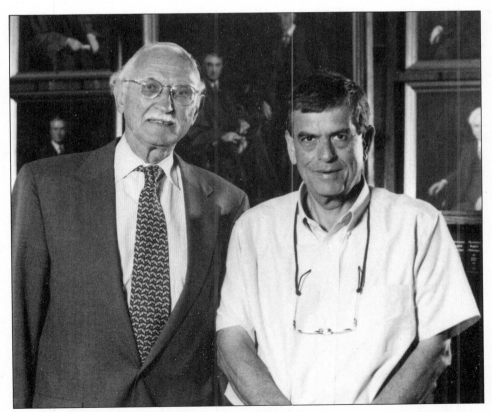

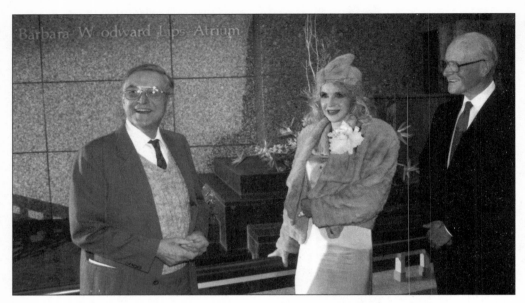

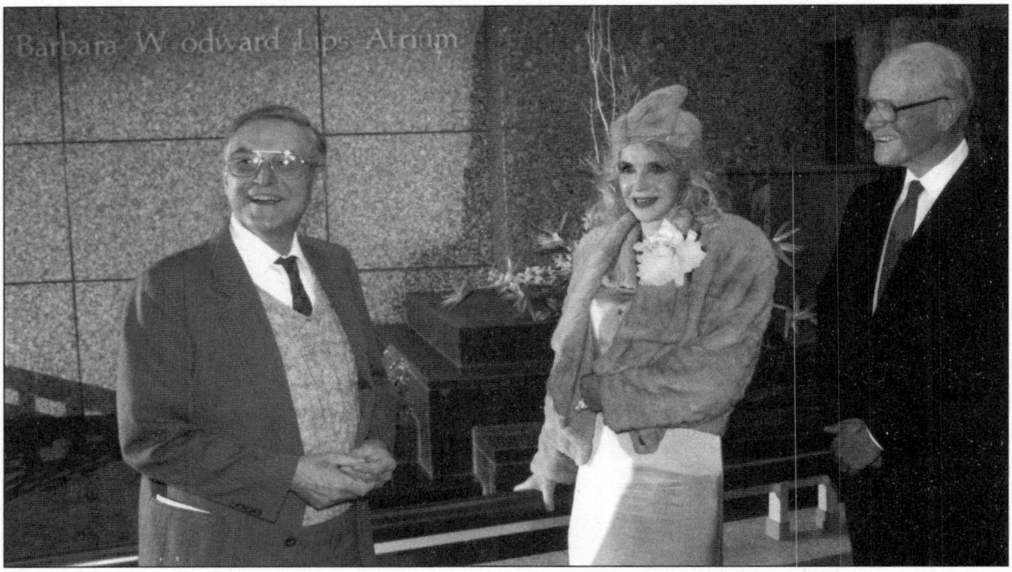

Mayo benefactor Barbara Woodward Lips, with Mayo physicians William McConahey (left) and Oliver Beahrs, in the atrium named for her in the Charlton Building. Her bequest of $127.9 million was the largest ever in Mayo history. (MAYO PHOTO ARCHIVES)

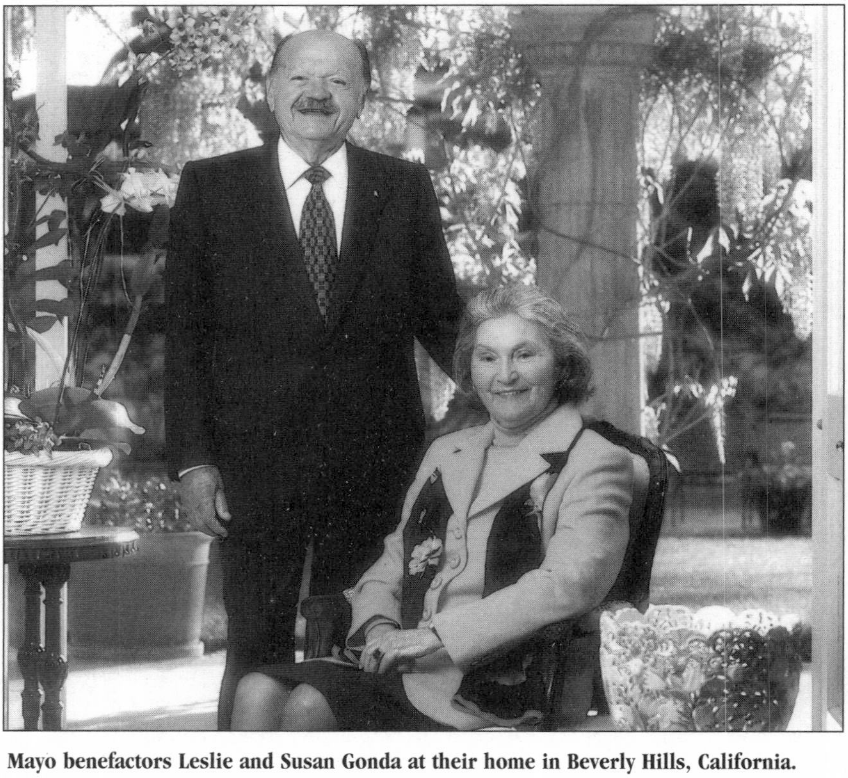

Mayo benefactors Leslie and Susan Gonda at their home in Beverly Hills, California.

Distinguished Mayo ophthalmologist Robert Waller, chair of the Mayo board of governors (left), thanks Leslie and Susan Gonda for providing major funding for the Gonda Vascular Center and later for the Gonda Building for integration of the Mayo Rochester medical practice. (MAYO PHOTO ARCHIVES)

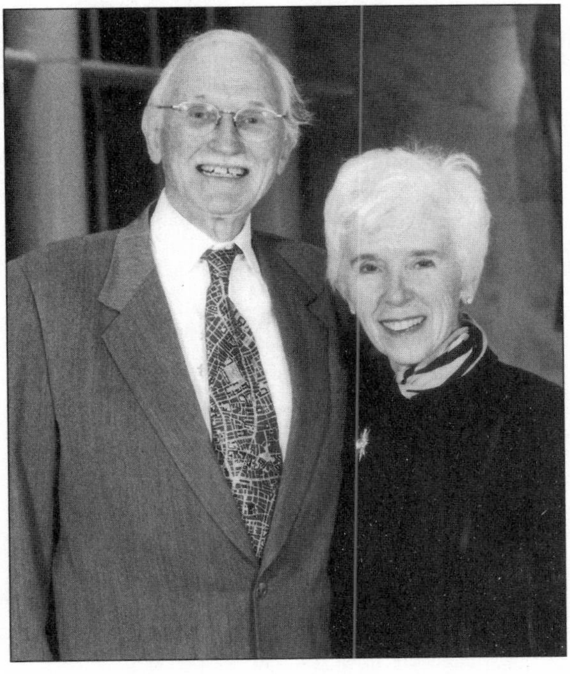

Marion and I attend the Gonda Building dedication in October 2001. (MAYO PHOTO ARCHIVES)

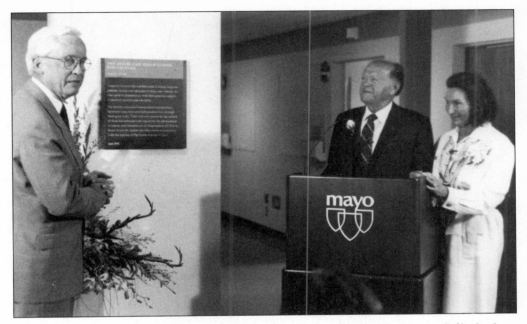

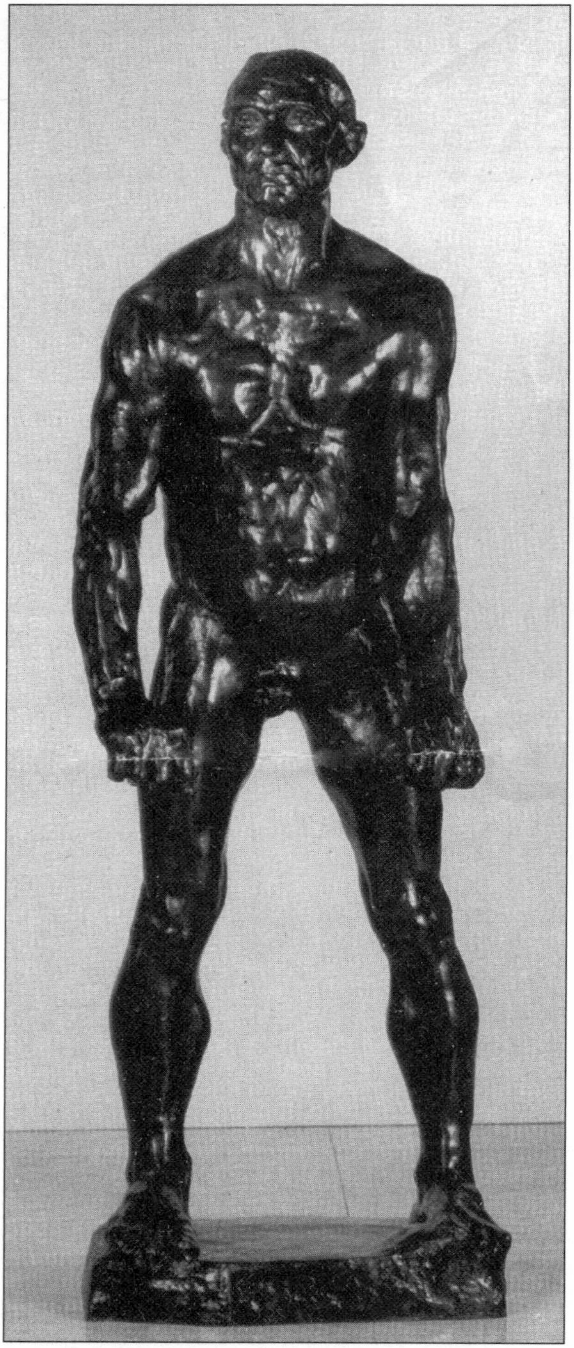

Auguste Rodin's *Jean d'Aire,* installed in the Siebens Building, was a gift from the Fran and Ray Stark Foundation in honor of E. Rolland Dickson, chair of the Mayo board of development. (MAYO PHOTO ARCHIVES)

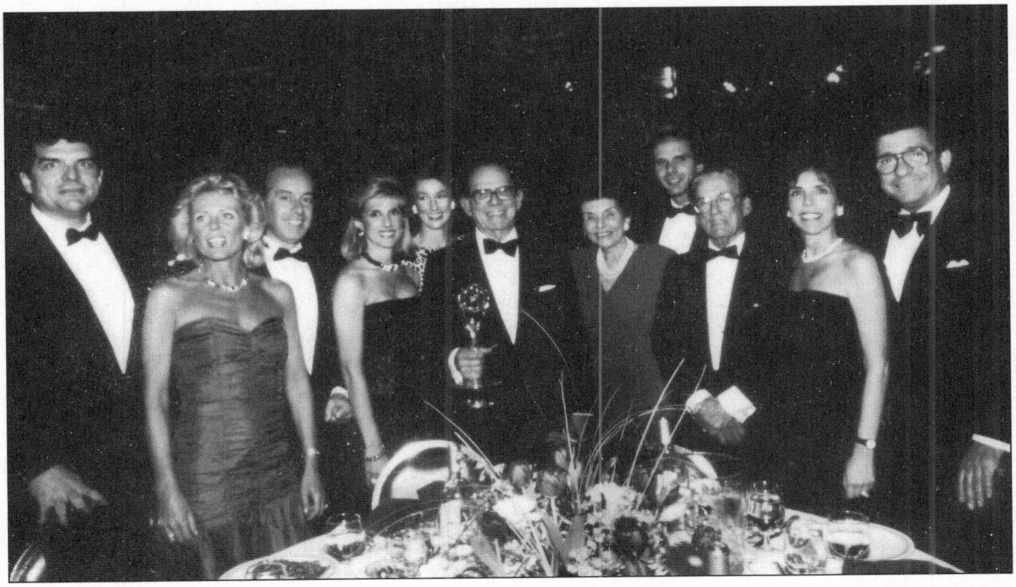

Goar Mestre (center) displays his Emmy, awarded him in 1987 for his contributions to broadcasting. His wife, Alicia, is on his left. My daughter, Gillian, is behind Goar; her husband, Eduardo Mestre, is behind and to the left of his mother.

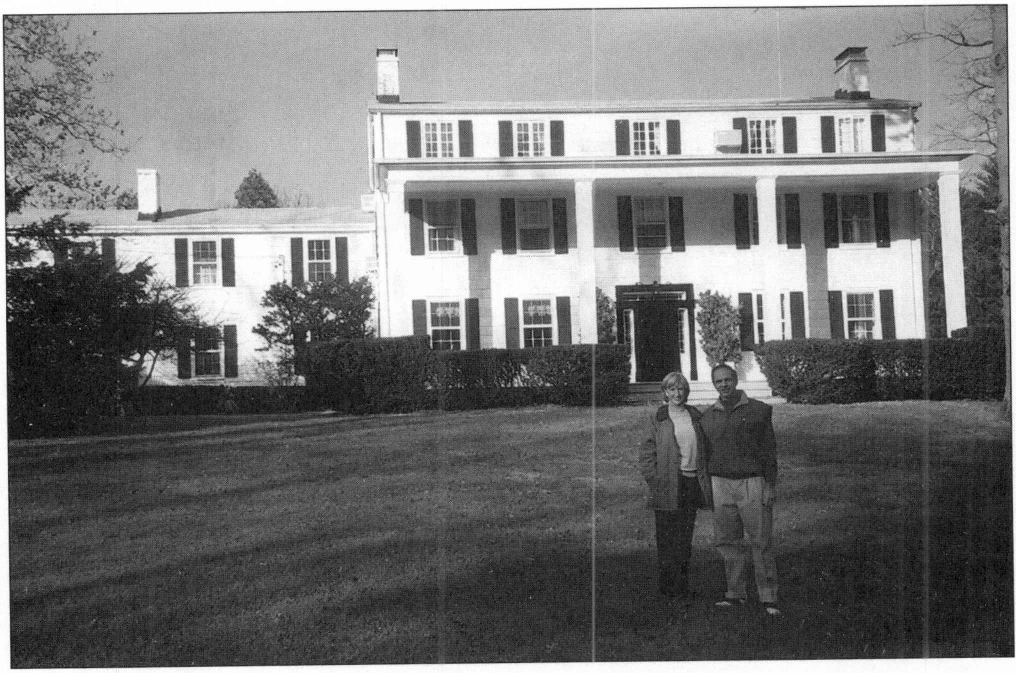

The home of my daughter and son-in-law, Gillian Shepherd and Eduardo Mestre, in Locust Valley, Long Island, New York.

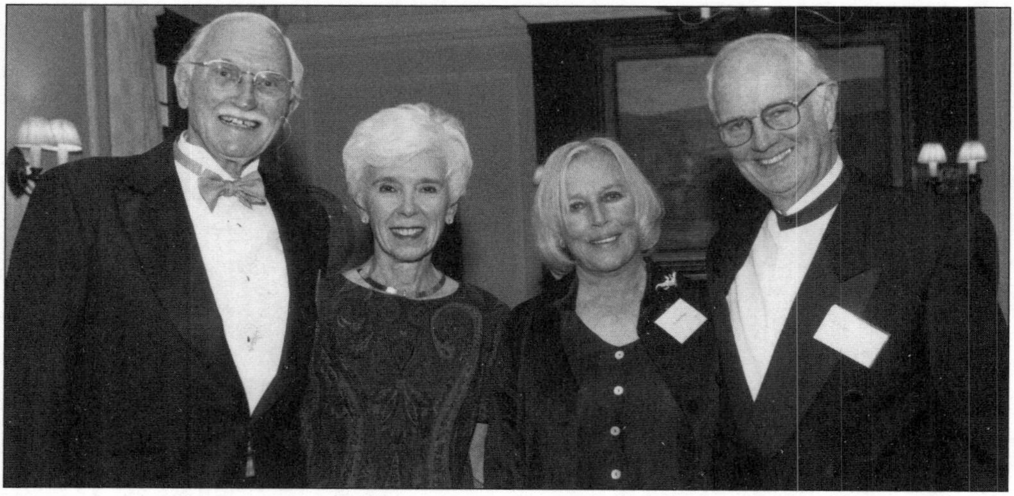

From left: Marion and I celebrate in May 2001 with Janet and B. Lawrence Riggs, honored as a Mayo Distinguished Alumnus for his studies of osteoporosis. (MAYO PHOTO ARCHIVES)

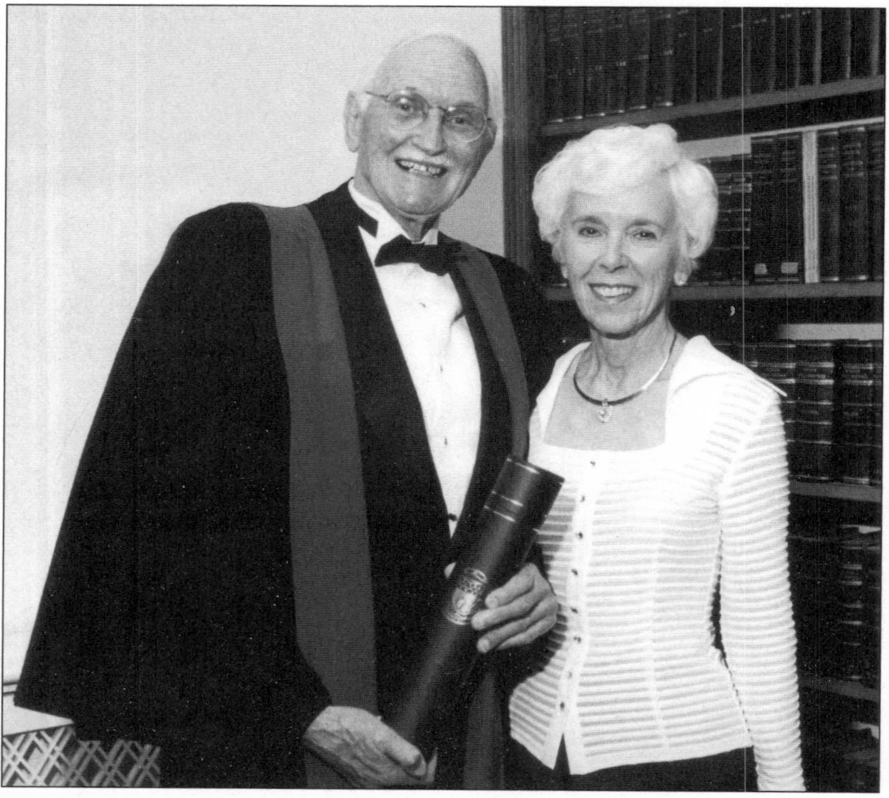

Marion and I traveled to Belfast in June 2003 when I became an honorary fellow of the Royal College of Physicians of Ireland.

Index

INDEX

This book was designed by

Mary Susan Oleson

Nashville, Tennessee

---

fonts used:

Florentine

and

Book Antiqua